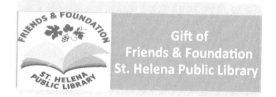

SANCTUARY

SANCTUARY

ESSENTIAL WISDOM *for* AN INSPIRED HOME

TONYA OLSEN

and

DEBONI SACRE

PLAIN SIGHT PUBLISHING

AN IMPRINT OF CEDAR FORT, INC.
SPRINGVILLE, UTAH

ISBN 13: 978-1-4621-1490-0

Published by Plain Sight Publishing, an imprint of Cedar Fort, Inc.
2373 W. 700 S., Springville, UT 84663
Distributed by Cedar Fort, Inc., www.cedarfort.com

LIBRARY OF CONGRESS CONTROL NUMBER: 2014956057

Cover and page design by Shawnda T. Craig
Cover design © 2015 by Lyle Mortimer
Edited by Eileen Leavitt

Printed in China

10 9 8 7 6 5 4 3 2 1

TABLE OF CONTENTS

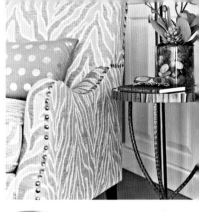

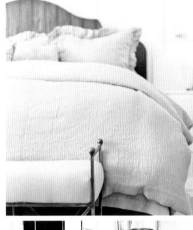
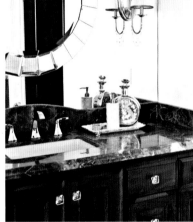
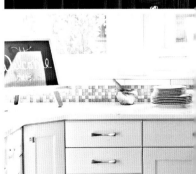

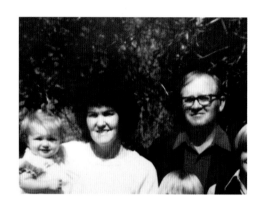

To my mom and dad,
who taught me what a sanctuary really is.

— Deboni

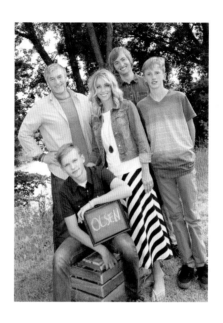

To my family, I love you.

—Tonya

ACKNOWLEDGMENTS

Sanctuary would not have been possible without the many people who assisted us in creating this book. First and foremost, Pamela Jensen—friend, colleague, and interior designer extraordinaire—thank you for investing your time, talent, knowledge, and expertise. We could not have done this without you.

Many thanks to the following:

Jenny Butler, Kristen Holm, and Samantha Zenger for keeping customers happy and business going during the many long days and hours; Cedar Fort for their support and guidance; and to our immediate family members for their patience, encouragement, and trust.

Introduction

INTRODUCTION

In the fall of 2011, I noticed a new store going in on the quaint main street of the suburban community where I currently live. Curious, I popped my head in the door to take a look. The smell of fresh paint and sawdust filled the air. As I glanced around, I saw pieces of furniture, tightly wrapped in cellophane and bubble wrap, strewn about the space. Shelves full of pillows and accessories lined the walls. Instantly, my pulse began to quicken at thought that this could be a new furniture store. Excitedly, I stepped further into the building and hollered a hello. In an instant, a petite blond popped out from a back room. "Hi! My name is Deboni. Can I help you?"

As Deboni (like *ebony* with a *d*) and I chatted, she explained that she was an interior designer and she was indeed opening a furniture store. If I remember our conversation correctly, I'm pretty sure I assaulted her on the spot and asked if she was looking for a business partner because, after all, I too was an interior designer and had always wanted to open my own store. Without a hint of being taken aback by my abrupt, forward approach, she responded, "Yes, actually, I am."

And that, my friends, is how Deboni and I met. I like to think of it as divine intervention. By the end of the week, we'd signed a contract, forged a partnership, and opened Liv Showroom, a full-service interior design firm and furniture showroom. Three years later, here we are.

Hi. Let me introduce myself. My name is Tonya Olsen. As you can probably guess, professionally, I am an interior designer, business owner, and author, just like Deboni. In the years we've practiced interior design (both together and on our own), we've had the honor and privilege of working with hundreds of great clients and have had the opportunity to design many fabulous spaces. In addition to our professional experience, we've also had years of personal experience building, renovating, and decorating our own homes for our own families.

We live in a world dictated by our physical senses. We see, touch, smell, taste, and hear the environment around us. Deboni and I have been trained to ensure the spaces we create are attractive, comfortable, and functional—all of which

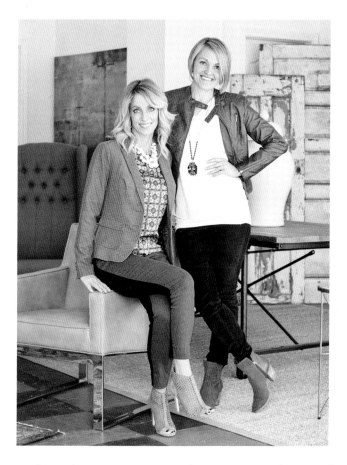

appeal to our physical senses. But great design is more than mechanics. Sure, there are basic design principles to consider, such as color, balance, proportion, and scale. These are the hard-and-fast rules that, when applied correctly, make the physical design of an interior successful. But what about the subtle, energetic elements within a space? The things less tangible? The things we can't see?

Every single one of us has been in a space that didn't feel quite right. It may have been professionally designed by a master architect and decorated with high-end finishes and expensive furniture. And yet, while we were unable to put our finger on it, something felt off-balance.

The fact of the matter is that our environments, particularly our homes, are made up of more than what we can see. They are filled with more than inanimate objects and serve more than to simply provide shelter. Our homes are where we eat, sleep, gather, and relax. Our homes are where we pray, contemplate, grow, and evolve. They are filled with memories, artifacts, history, and spirit. Our homes are where we truly live.

Don't get me wrong. I like pretty things just as much as the next person. I'm always poring over magazines and scouring the Internet for the latest and greatest interior design trends. It's what I do for a living. But Deboni and I understand on a deeper level that our homes represent a physical manifestation of our personal selves. The thoughts, feelings, and emotions within a home are as important as, if not more important than, what a home looks like.

So what makes a home a sanctuary? We believe an inspired home is made up of four essential components: physical, mental, emotional, and spiritual. Each component is interconnected and, when in balance, creates harmony. It's kind of like creating heaven on earth or combining our dreams with reality.

If you're like most of us, you probably won't be able to tackle every element of your sanctuary all at once. That means very possibly living with spaces that either don't function perfectly or don't uplift you quite the way you prefer. But creating a plan for the overall space is key. If you have a plan in place for how your home will function and inspire you in the future, you'll be able to handle the temporary imperfections.

Focus on more than how your space will look. Consider how your space will function on a day-to-day basis. You must take your entire home into consideration, including the exterior living spaces. Your home is a multifaceted organism, and each part contributes to the whole. Assessing your storage needs will go a long way in the functionality of your home. Ask a friend or family member for their thoughts on the functionality of your home. An outside opinion can give you a fresh perspective when you are stuck with a particular design dilemma.

As we'll recommend later in the book, once you have your hopes, dreams, and aspirations on paper, figure out where you can realistically start. Start with one room or one area if that's all you can do. The point is, just get started. If you're not aware of how your environment affects you, you'll quickly see after just completing even a small portion how much the feeling in your space will change. One change will eventually lead to another, and before you know it, your entire space will be transformed into the sanctuary you've been dreaming of.

Deboni and I believe that our homes are the most sacred places on earth. Through experience and inspiration, our goal in writing this book is to share what we've learned: practical ideas, shared knowledge, and essential wisdom about how you can create an inspired home.

HOW THIS BOOK WORKS

Sanctuary is broken down into four parts featuring favorite projects created by Liv Showroom and how they relate to the physical, mental, emotional, and spiritual elements of a space. Our clients graciously opened their homes and visited with us about their lifestyles, decorating purposes, and personal insights into their spaces.

Part 1, STRUCTURE, addresses the physical portion of a space, including walls, floors, and ceilings, and how their configuration relates to the occupants of the home. This includes human scale, gathering spaces, and private or in-between spaces.

Part 2, ATMOSPHERE, covers the mental components of space, including light and sound, color and design principles, and organization or order.

Part 3, EXPRESSION, showcases emotional aspects of space, such as personality, details and materials, and things that matter.

Part 4, REFLECTION, presents symbolism in our environments, places for introspection, and how a space connects to nature and spirituality.

At the end of each part, we've pulled together additional elements within each space in a section called "Tying It Together: Elements of a Sacred Space." These pages display how various components of structure, atmosphere, expression, and reflection work together to create a sanctuary within each featured room.

But before that, it's important to know how to create an interior design plan and budget. In "Words of Wisdom," we cover the basics of getting started, moving forward, and paying for your project. Throughout the book, Deboni and I give simple yet profound advice to live by. We adhere to these straightforward, time-honored principles in both our work and our personal lives.

Finally, Deboni and I have provided you with a list of our favorite resources for shopping. Most of the items featured in each project were purchased from one of our recommended retailers.

Regardless of your style or budget, our sincerest hope is that you'll use this book as an inspiration and guide for creating a sanctuary in your own home.

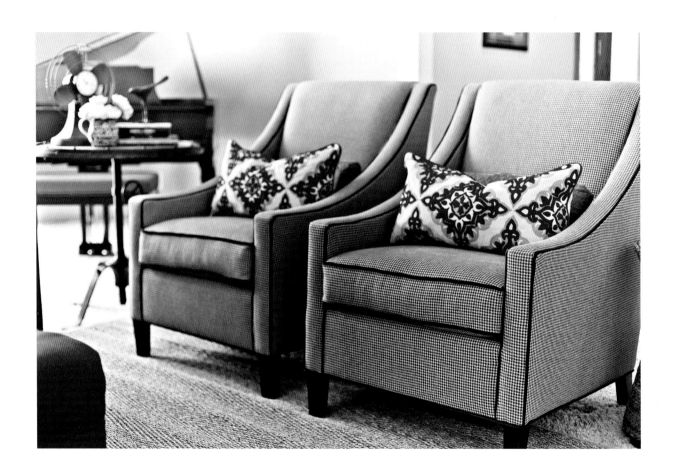

WORDS OF WISDOM

If you don't think planning is important, think again. At least some form of planning is paramount to the success of your project, especially when consciously creating your sanctuary.

Throughout our years of experience, we've noticed consistent and essential components of undertaking an interior design project. No matter the size of the project, it makes sense to be aware and to put into practice the following words of wisdom:

CREATE A WISH LIST

The desire to create is human nature, and our homes are the most obvious place to leave our mark. A true sanctuary possesses the unlimited potential of our ability to create. That doesn't necessarily translate to spending lots of money; it simply means making the absolute most of what we realistically have to work with.

When building a wish list, indulge yourself, and let your imagination run wild. If money were no object, allow yourself to envision all the features, finishes, and flourishes you'd like to see in your space. Think outside the box, and consider what you'd normally see as a risk. Write down everything you'd like to do and buy, even if it seems unrealistic. You never know what is obtainable with a little creativity. This is what makes interior design is so fun—imagining the possibilities.

Now that you've unleashed your fantasies, reel them in according to the meaningful intentions of your family and lifestyle. You may have always wanted a two-island kitchen with commercial appliances and seating for twelve, but if your home realistically won't accommodate such an extravagance, tailor your needs to what you can work with. For example, if a sixty-inch freestanding Wolf range won't fit in your space or your budget, consider a smaller range that fulfills the same cooking requirements but costs a lot less. Instead of double islands, consider where you might tuck in a small prep area, and create ways to work in additional seating. Have fun, but don't forget to be practical.

GATHER INSPIRATION

Gather images of rooms you like. Our sanctuaries come to life when we fill them with the things we love. Looking at pictures gives us an idea of what might be possible, not only creatively but also pragmatically.

There are many fantastic websites that offer inspiration and ways of keeping your favorite ideas organized. Houzz and Pinterest are the two most popular sites for interior design ideas, but don't forget to consider other sources as well. Books, magazines, and blogs offer a wealth of resources that you might not have considered.

Take your time while collecting your ideas. Personal taste evolves over time, and what you thought was a fabulous idea one day will more than likely change over weeks and months. Remember, tastes change much more frequently than budget typically allows.

GAIN PERSPECTIVE

Take a step back and detach yourself from your space. As interior designers and homeowners, we can testify that the hardest jobs for us are the ones that are personal. Taking an objective look and assessing the reality of an interior design project can provide creative and practical solutions we might not otherwise have considered. When we enter a space from an outside perspective, it's easier to look at it logically rather than emotionally.

Ask yourself some questions. What do you like about it? What do you dislike? What activities happen here? Is your home efficient, practical, and organized? How comfortable is your home for your lifestyle? What do you want your home to look and feel like?

Don't forget to consider others living in your home. A spouse and other family members may outwardly appear not have an interest, but realistically they often have very specific opinions. A sanctuary is a sacred space encompassing the considerations of each and every occupant.

At the beginning of each part in, we've included some soul-searching questions to examine. Really take the time to consider the reality of yourself, your family, and your lifestyle. Be open to all the possibilities, but also be willing to compromise.

PRIORITIZE

Remember, Rome wasn't built in a day. Although it's not impossible, it is usually unrealistic to have an unlimited budget and the ability to do everything at once. Breaking down your projects into phases and completing them over a period of time, whether it's days, weeks, or months, is usually the best way to go. If you can't afford to do it all at once, don't. Moving forward a little bit at a time, within your financial means, is a vital and underlying component of creating a sanctuary.

Consider which rooms or projects are top priorities. Typically, the main living area, including the entry, and gathering spaces such as the living room and kitchen are the best places to start. Once these rooms are established, the completed design can influence the rest of the house.

Be realistic about the time frame. More often than not, projects take longer than we initially anticipate. While painting a small bedroom over a weekend is probably doable, renovating a kitchen will more than likely take months. Expect delays, snags, and surprises. If you're special ordering specialty items, it often takes several weeks to fulfill an order. It's helpful to break down and itemize the list of work to be done.

DRAFT YOUR DESIGN BLUEPRINT

Put it on paper and on purpose. Even a simple outline or plan is better than nothing at all. Once it's written on paper, it's easier to turn it into reality, and it will help keep you on track.

Sketching out potential design options is a great way to brainstorm solutions you might not otherwise have considered. Try visualizing different furniture of various sizes and shapes. Factor in the basic elements of design, including scale, proportion, and size. The elements of a sanctuary always result in harmony and balance.

DO YOUR RESEARCH

Are you willing and able to do it yourself? How complex is the project, and what skills do you have in realistically in being able to tackle it? Can you afford an interior designer or contractor? Are they trained, knowledgeable, and experienced? Do they have a license? What have others said about their quality of work? A home won't become a sanctuary if it's riddled with problems that could have been avoided with a little time and research.

CREATE A BUDGET

If only we had unlimited financial means to fulfill our wildest dreams, right? But decorating on a budget isn't about being cheap; it's about being smart. An astronomical budget isn't the only means to a successful end. When creating a sanctuary, making informed decisions will always give you the best value for your money.

Understanding the costs of labor and merchandise will go a long way in determining your budget. If you haven't shopped for a new sofa in twenty years, be prepared for some sticker shock. A quality sofa can start in price around $1,000 or more. Labor and services typically range from hourly to square footage pricing.

Be sure to factor in the unpredictable. Socking away an additional fifteen to twenty percent of your budget will alleviate stress when unexpected expenses pop up. And they always do.

It's good to invest in your home. Fancy vacations and expensive getaways are nice, but how often do we really get to do those? Consider your home as the place you escape to each day. Your sanctuary is the best place to invest in for the best day-to-day retreat money can buy.

Invest in big-ticket items such as quality furniture, permanent features, an extraordinary focal point, or items you'll use every day. Splurging on items that hold or add value is always a good investment.

However, don't confuse value with worth. If you travel and like to collect mementos, especially items you'll put on display, it may be worth it to spend a little more for the sentimental significance it will lend over a lifetime. Spend less on trendy, knickknack items such as pillows and other decorative accessories. These items come and go with the changing times and can easily and inexpensively be updated. Be wary of impulse buying. It's easy to get off track financially during the process. Homes filled with unnecessary and whimsical purchases become cluttered easily, and unnecessary clutter will quickly turn your sanctuary into a space that is confining and untidy.

Finally, take a look around at the things you already have. Rather than spending money on new things, go through your home and consider new uses for old items. Look at outdated items with a fresh perspective. You'd be surprised what you can create with even a modest budget, simple planning, and basic design skills. When creating your sanctuary, be ever vigilant with following your budget.

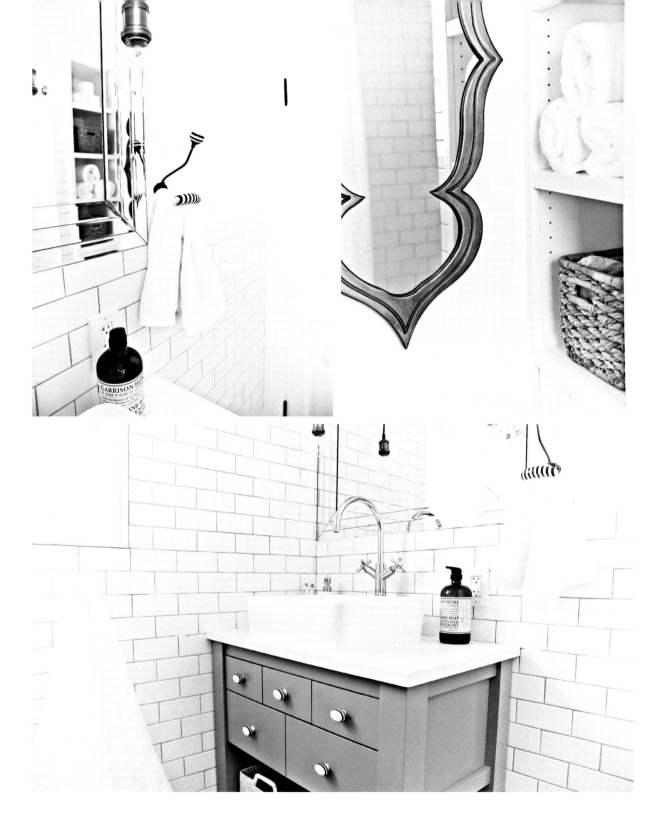

ELEMENTS OF A SANCTUARY

Since the dawn of man, societies of every kind have intuitively understood the sacredness of architecture and our innate connection to our environment. Humans have always been sensitive to their surroundings as a primal need to survive. You were born with an inherent awareness of your environment. Although we may not be conscious of it, this awareness exists in all of us. Whether you have realized it before or not, that's why your home and the way it's designed is integral to your physical, mental, emotional, and spiritual well-being.

In recent years, there's been a palpable shift in what we long for in home design. We've discovered that bigger is not necessarily better. Rather than building larger, we're building smarter. Architect Sarah Susanka kick-started a movement in residential home design when she released *The Not So Big House: A Blueprint for the Way We Really Live* in 1998. Sarah's design philosophy focuses on quality rather than quantity and maximizing the full functional potential of smaller spaces. When we live in a quality-based environment, it influences our well-being.

We are at a tipping point in history where we long for our homes to reflect the balance between mortality and divinity, purpose and practicality. We innately long

to feel stable, safe, and secure
to feel a sense of belonging and be part of a community
to have privacy and time to reflect
to have choice and control
to be creative and expressive
to have a sense of status and achievement
to understand the meaning of life
to connect to nature

The bottom line is that we want to feel at home both in our houses and in our lives, and we try to do this by changing the things we are aware of—the things we assume must be the problem, such as not having enough space and time. But some problems are less visible; they're about qualities rather than quantities, so they are more difficult to identify, articulate, and resolve. We can't create more of a sense of home if we don't understand where that feeling comes from. When a home is consciously infused with these properties, it becomes a sanctuary. It is essential that we create for ourselves, and for our planet, an inspired home.

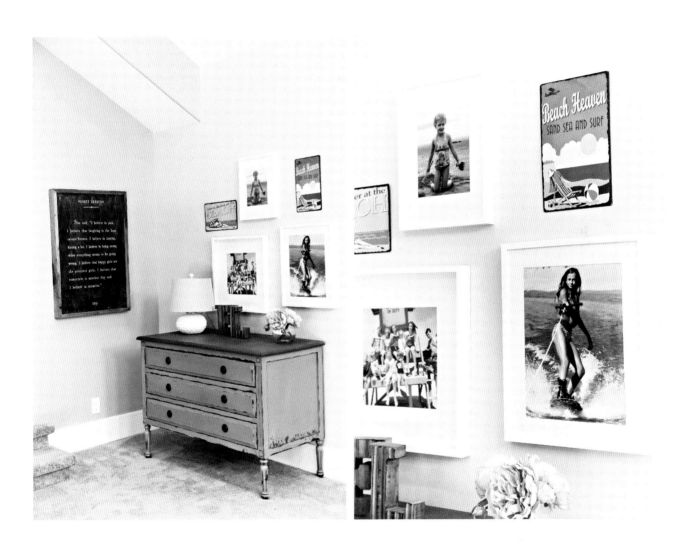

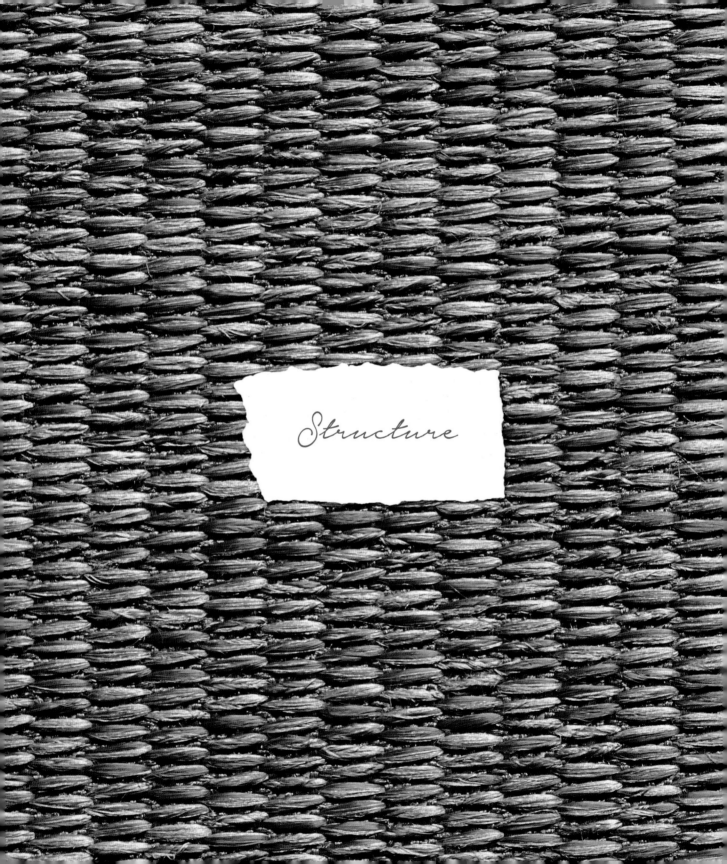

Structure

STRUCTURE

As humans, we have an innate awareness of our environment. At a primal level, all humans long for safety, security, and comfort.

The physical structure of a home is determined by a combination of its architectural elements. It's where the walls, ceilings, and floors meet to create our physical reality. The structure of our home satisfies our primal needs by providing shelter and keeping us safe. The structure of our homes is divided into functional and efficient spaces such as kitchens, living rooms, bedrooms, and bathrooms. These spaces can be public, private, or both. The structure of our home sets the tone for the rest of the house, so it's important to give thought to how it influences and inspires.

The physical attributes of our home influence our family and group safety and security, ability to provide for life's necessities, feeling at home, familial law, and order.

Our physical space is where human ergonomics (that's a fancy word for knowing how we best function in relation to our environment) plays an important role. A well-designed space will fulfill all of our practical needs. While the structure itself is not what makes a home sacred, the important elements of the structure must work cohesively to support our lifestyle. The way we experience life has much to do with the structure of our home.

More than simply providing physical shelter and safety for our families and belongings, a house must meet our emotional needs for shelter and safety, creating the feeling of safety and protection. Protecting you from the elements is only part of the purpose of a well-designed structure. In today's modern world, with things coming at us from every direction, we need that landing zone to draw our families and friends together. A sanctuary does not simply fulfill our physical needs of protection. It also fulfills our mental, emotional, and spiritual needs.

Our rooms are meant to accommodate activity. A well-designed sanctuary lends focus to the lifestyle of the inhabitants. The structure becomes the focus of life at home. Some of this activity is shared, and some of it is private.

An inspired home balances gathering and private spaces according to the needs and desired lifestyle goals of the inhabitants. It has good flow and scale of rooms that simply *feel* good.

Human Scale

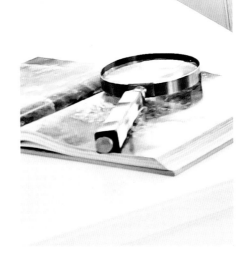

"Man knows that the world is not made on a human scale; and he wishes that it were."

—André Malraux

HUMAN SCALE

Intuitively, we know what feels good in a space. Physically, mentally, emotionally, and spiritually, we feel good in a space that is well-designed in its proportion and flow of parts. Good design and layout has a sense of harmony. This harmony in flow and function creates an emotional stillness.

Harmony, proportion, and balance are the building blocks of basic design principles that affect us in regard to our environment. A home designed with human scale in mind aligns proportionately with the functionality of our human physical characteristics.

Scale and proportion are the most important of the principles. Some proportional relationships are more pleasing than others and offer a certain comfort level. The ancient Greeks discovered the Golden Section, which sought to reduce all proportion to a simple formula: the ratio of the smaller section to the larger section should be the same as that of the larger section to the whole. Scale, in residential design especially, is most appropriate when it complements and easily accommodates the average human form. When scale and proportion are "off," the room feels uncomfortable.

Interior Reflection

ASK YOURSELF THE FOLLOWING QUESTIONS WHEN CONTEMPLATING
THE **PHYSICAL STRUCTURE** OF YOUR HOME:

1. How can my home best support myself, my family, and my guests?

2. Do I utilize all of the space in my existing home?

3. Are there spaces I can convert to make them multifunctional?

4. Do I often have guests, and if so, how many? How often?
Do they stay for an extended period of time?

5. How important is privacy? Do I need a quiet place to contemplate, study, or work?

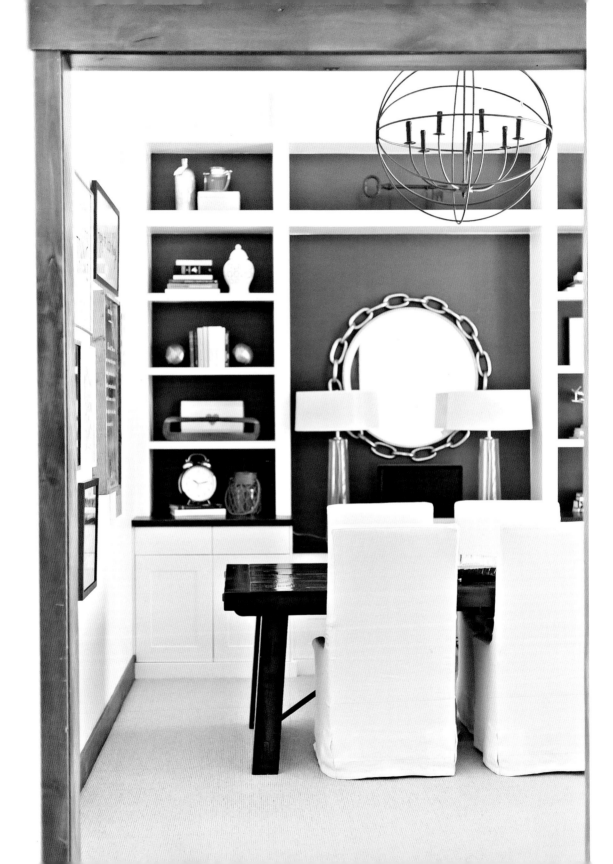

INSPIRATION POINT

Renovating a dark, underused, high-ceilinged room into a comfortable, multi-functional space near her home's entry was Lisa Taggart's goal. The mother of three called on interior designer Pamela Jensen to help design an office not only for her, but also for her kids to do homework and art projects.

Lisa wanted the room to feel cozier, so Pamela designed floor-to-ceiling built-in bookshelves, painting them the same color as the ceiling and contrasting the back wall with a defining color. The hard-working shelves serve two contrasting functions: concealing storage and displaying personal treasures.

Pamela further enhanced the intimate feeling of the space by adding a dark-stained, chunky table in the center of the room. The mass and size of the table is proportionate to the room without making the space feel cramped. The rustic nature of the table is the perfect place for Lisa's kids to do homework and art projects. Slipcovered chairs soften the room and can easily be washed if necessary.

The thoughtful planning and detailed design gives the room a comfortable, fresh, and sophisticated look.

MISTAKES
TRYING

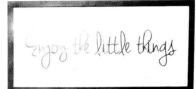
enjoy the little things

IF YOU
WANT IT
WORK
FOR IT
"it's that simple"

You are never too old to Dream a New Dream

DALAI LAMA

He said, "There are only two days in the year that nothing can be done. One is called *yesterday* and the other is called *tomorrow*, so today is the right day to love, believe, do and mostly live."

54.

IF YOU
CAN BE
ANYTHING
be kind

"HOW you
MAKE OTHERS FEEL
ABOUT THEMSELVES,
SAYS A LOT
ABOUT YOU."

WHATEVER YOU
decide to do
MAKE SURE IT
MAKES YOU
Happy

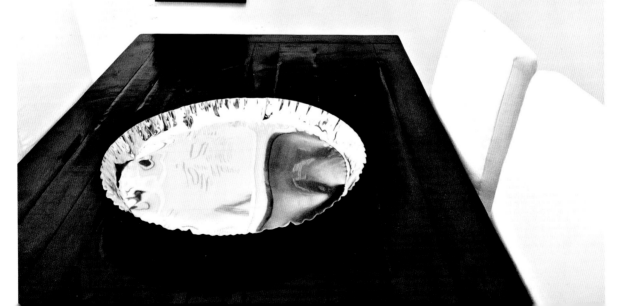

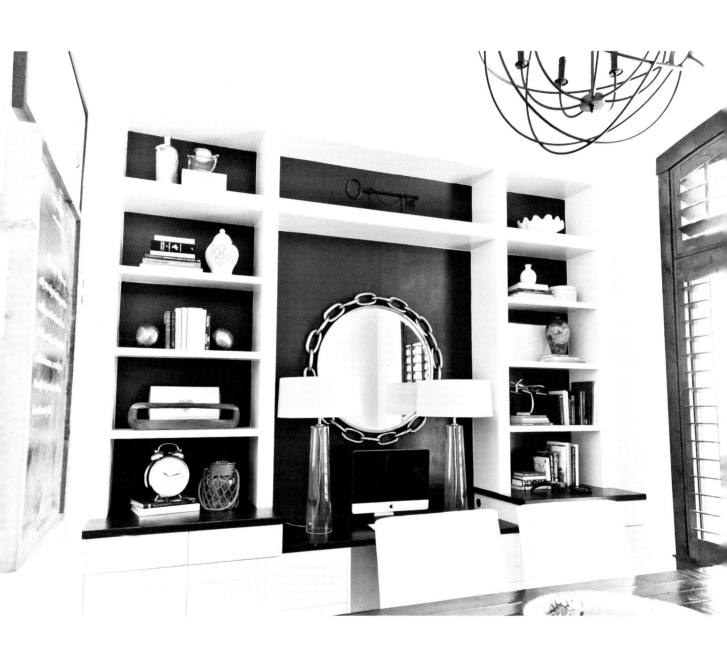

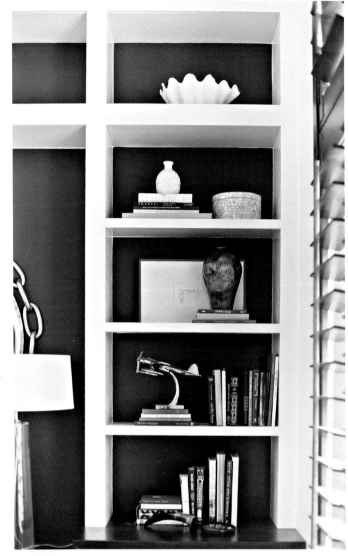

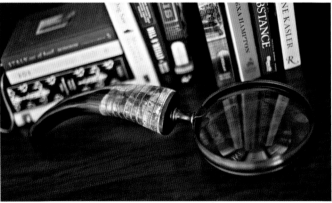

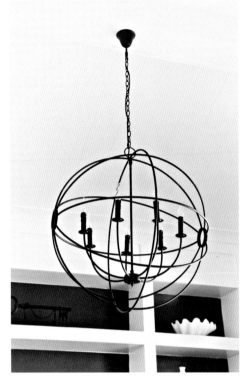

TO VISUALLY ADD height to the room and avoid awkward unused space, Pamela designed the built-in bookshelves to go to the ceiling. She opted to keep the back of the bookshelves painted a smokey gray-blue, which adds contrast and makes it visually recede.

ESPRESSO-STAINED WALNUT adds character and warmth to the built-in bookshelves while highlighting the Taggart's collectibles.

TONGUE AND GROOVE flanks a center beam, creating subtle detail on the ceiling. Introducing the over-sized scale of a large orb chandelier proportionately fills the space while creating visual interest.

TYING IT TOGETHER

Elements of a Sanctuary

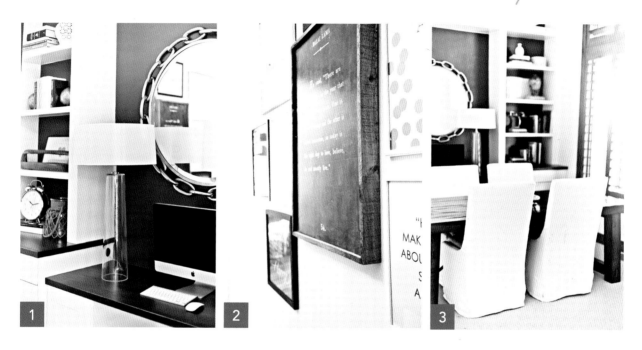

1. CLEAN EDGES, STRAIGHT lines, and minimal detailing give these built-ins a contemporary yet traditional vibe. Layering *things that matter* on the shelves and adding a mirror to the back wall create character and depth.

2. LISA CHOSE TO create a gallery wall of her favorite motivational quotes. The creative collection adds a touch of whimsy while providing daily reminders of *inspiration*.

3. THIS OFFICE IS designed with multiple seats as a place for the whole family to *gather* for games and other family or school activities.

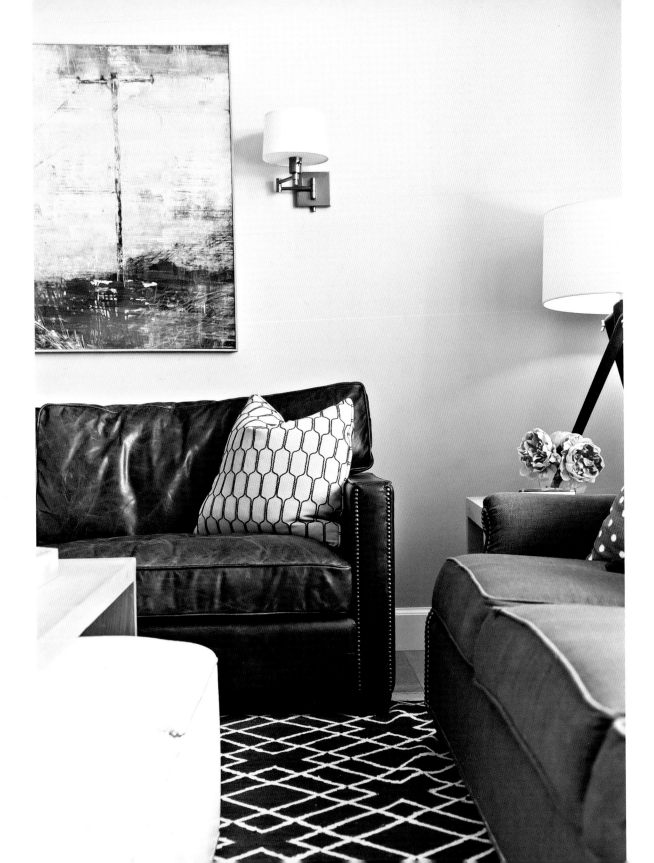

A FRESH START

Interior designer Deboni Sacre can certainly relate to the age-old adage "The cobbler's kids don't have shoes." Spending the past three years focusing her time, energy, and finances on her business, Liv Showroom, had left the interior of her own home neglected and borderline shabby. She knew something needed to change.

Deboni and her husband purchased their home in the early years of their marriage and hadn't planned on staying there for long. Ten years and four children later, the Sacre family decided they're at home—for the long haul. In addition, volunteering her own home to be featured in *Sanctuary* was the extra push she needed to take action in her own space.

And take action she did. Deboni created a plan to remodel her entry and living room, the two main areas seen upon entering her house. In the original design of the home, the two areas lacked separation and identity. Awkward angles and multiple ceiling heights made the space feel uncomfortable.

The new design seamlessly blends the two areas together while giving them their own distinct character. By adding detailed millwork and uniform ceiling height, the overall space is cohesive. Navy, fuchsia, and teal introduce a playful color palette to create a lively gathering space for this growing family.

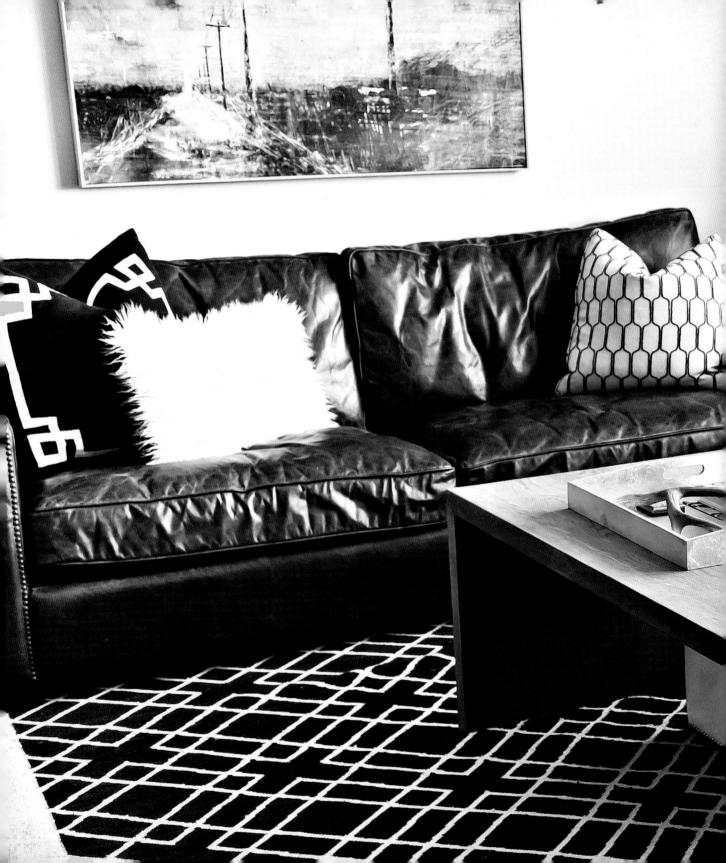

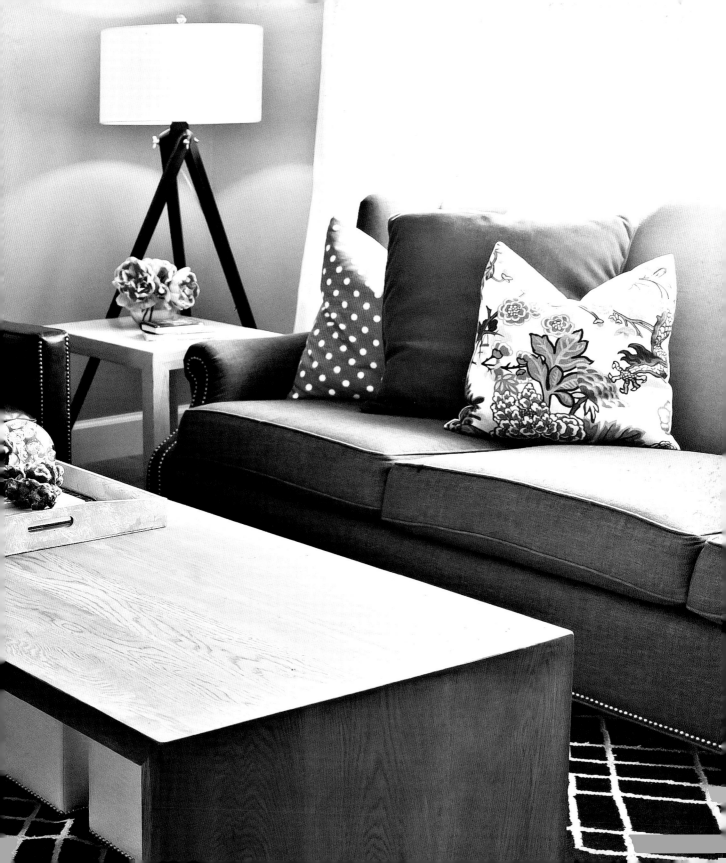

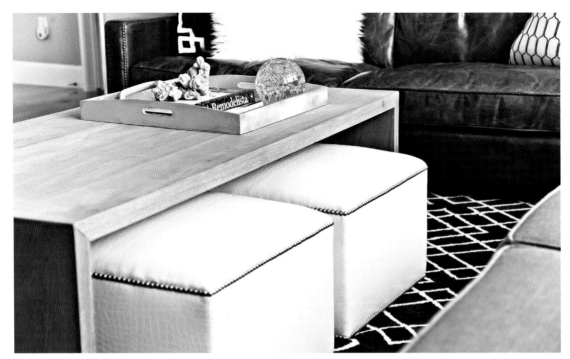

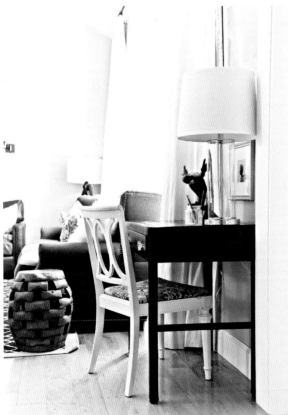

A CUSTOM-DESIGNED coffee table is functional and versatile. Deboni fashioned the piece to be streamlined and durable. Leather ottomans conveniently tuck underneath when they're not used for lounging or additional seating. A decorative tray serves to corral remotes and children's books, and it doubles as a coaster for holding drinks.

A FRAMED OPENING was added to the threshold between the living room and kitchen. The simple detail serves as a buffer zone and creates separation from the living room. A cozy desk provides an area for homework.

TYING IT TOGETHER

Elements of a Sanctuary

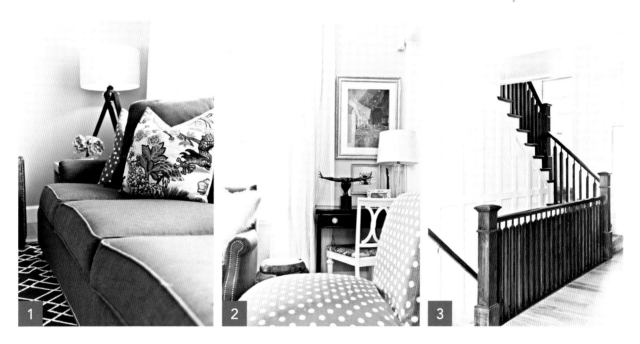

1 THE LENGTH OF A SOFA should always be proportionate to the size and *scale* of the room. Here, an extra-long sofa fills the space while maximizing seating.

2 FUCHSIA POLKA-DOT CHAIRS add *personality* to this *gathering space*. White, floor-to-ceiling window panels soften imposing windows.

3 A CEILING BRIDGE was added to create separation between the entry and living room. Conversely, finish detail like board-and-batten was added to the stairway wall to tie the rooms together.

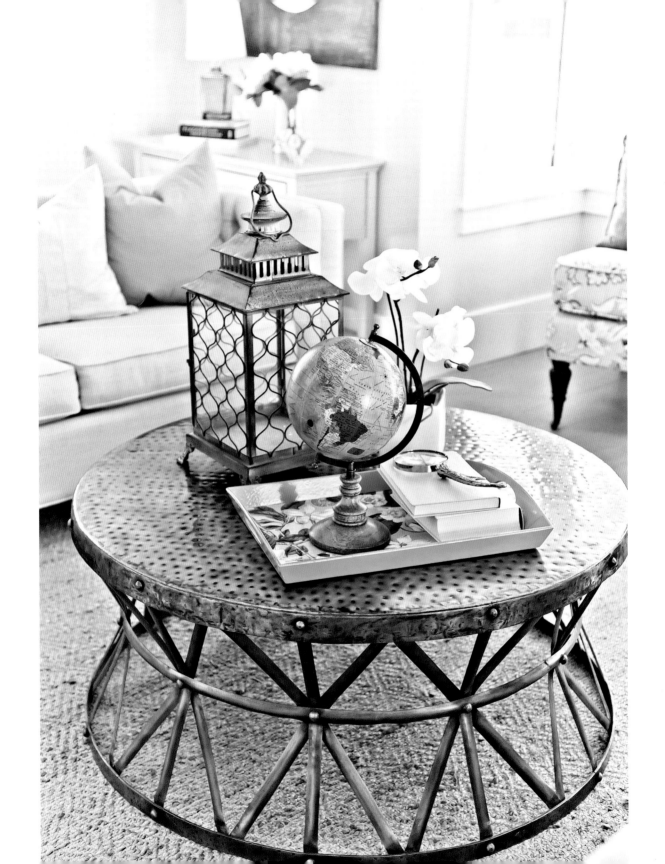

LET ME ENTERTAIN YOU

Not every home has a personal story to tell . . . yet. But it's not hard to imagine this model home as a potential sanctuary. Designer Tonya Olsen designed this tranquil haven on the shore of a community lake for homebuilder Rainey Homes.

This model is named "The Entertainer" for good reason. The main level was consciously designed to include large windows and numerous sets of french doors, which open to a wraparound patio. Soft hues in various shades of turquoise, green, and blue meander throughout the open living space and carry the "lake" theme from room to room.

Although the dining and living room are essentially one room, small details, such as a built-in cabinet installed directly between each space, create separation and a comfortable sense of proportion. Varying ceiling heights and architectural details from room to room further create a sense of division and influence our inherent sense of human scale.

Likely homebuyers, or those simply looking for inspiration, can surely envision a future sanctuary in this one-of-a-kind home.

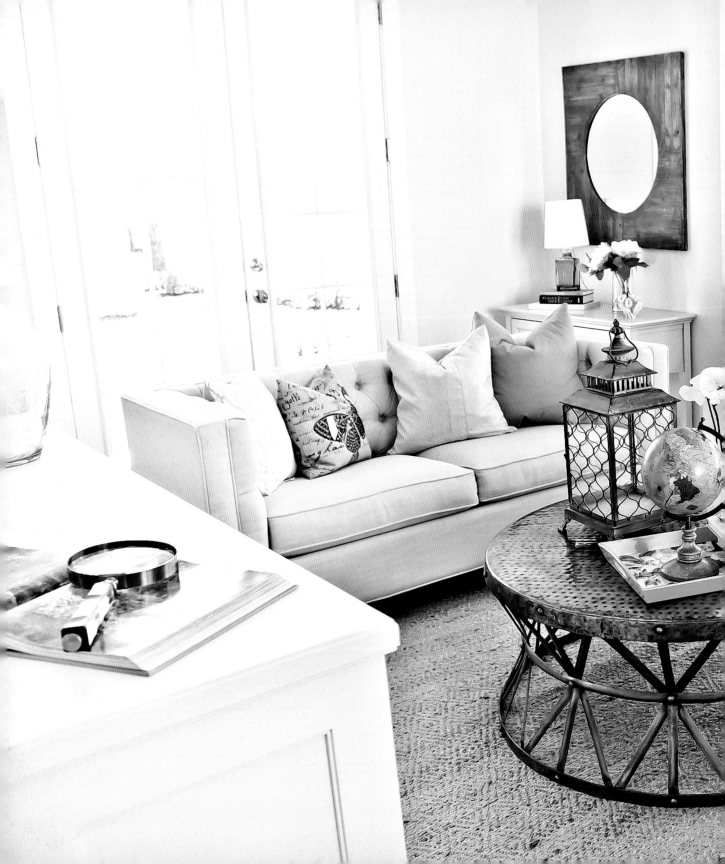

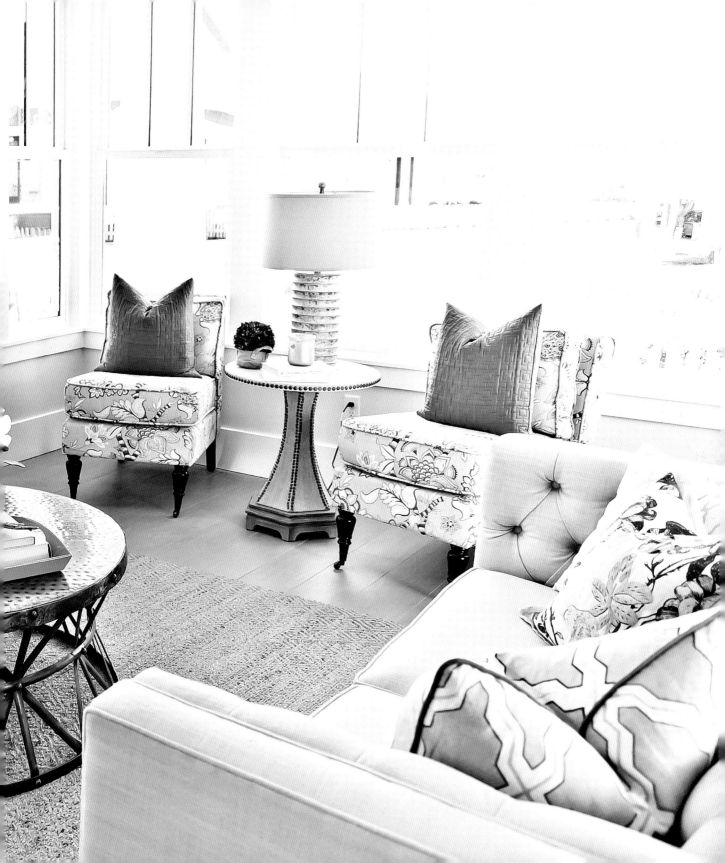

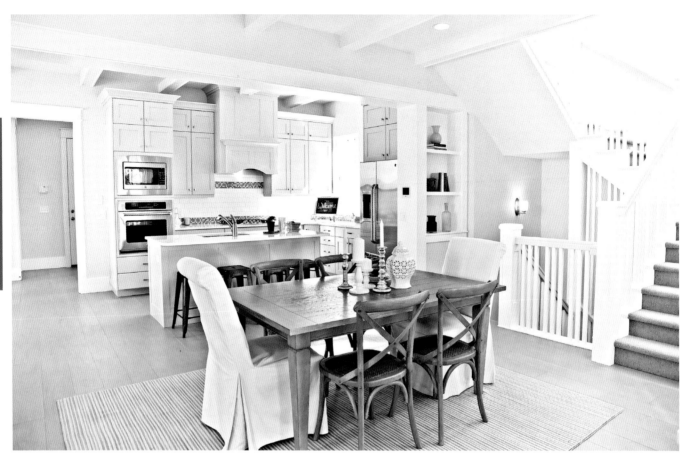

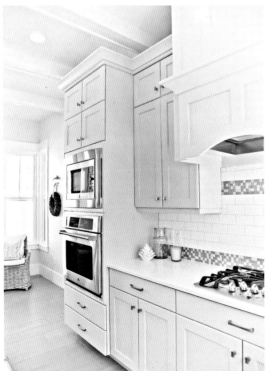

AN OPEN FLOOR plan is the ideal home design for entertaining. The kitchen is separate, yet part of the dining room, providing plenty of seating for family and friends.

THE KITCHEN CABINETS were painted a robin-egg blue to introduce a vibrant yet subtle splash of color. A double band of colorful mosaic tiles intersect rows of white subway tile on the backsplash. The delightful color scheme is inviting yet relaxing for large groups of people.

PORCELAIN CREATED to look like natural wood flooring gives a natural and clean look to the space.

TYING IT TOGETHER
Elements of a Sanctuary

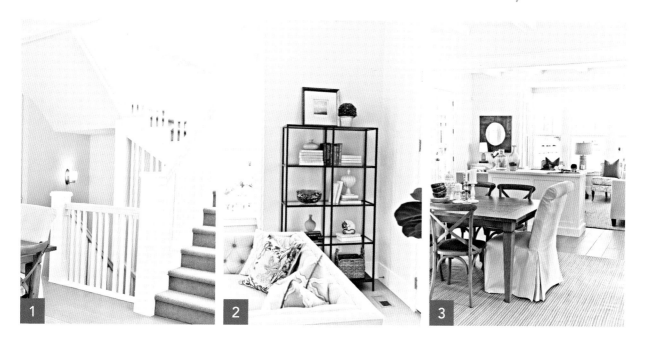

1 THE HANDRAIL was painted the same buoyant blue as the kitchen cabinets. This creative *detail* links the two spaces together while pulling the color throughout the house.

2 AN OPEN AND AIRY étagère displays a collection of *things that matter*, such as artwork, books, and other accessories.

3 A COZY NOOK, adjacent to the kitchen, creates the perfect *in-between space*. A set of chairs and a small side table provide intimate seating for two.

Gathering Spaces

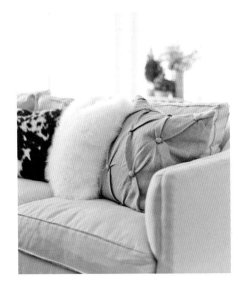

"Furnish your room for conversation and the
chairs will take care of themselves."

—Sibyl Colefax

GATHERING SPACES

A well-designed gathering space is rich with functionality and style. A gathering space is more than just a space for entertaining. The interior design of an environment can facilitate or discourage social interaction. For example, an inviting space with comfortable seating encourages family and friends to stay and visit.

Gathering spaces are the places within our home where we can connect with one another, help each other, and simply enjoy being with each other. For this reason, we are physically, mentally, emotionally, and spiritually supported through the gathering spaces in our homes.

Gathering rooms are places of activity and places of movement from the core of the home to more private spaces. Every home should have a clear "heart" of the home. This heart should be generous and attractive so that it's in the main circulation of traffic. It is a place that everyone passes by.

This is the place of connection for the household members. We need human contact in our lives, so this heart of the home is essential to our well-being.

Every sanctuary deserves at least one functional yet flexible space for gathering friends and family. After all, to you, your home is one of the most significant gathering places in the world.

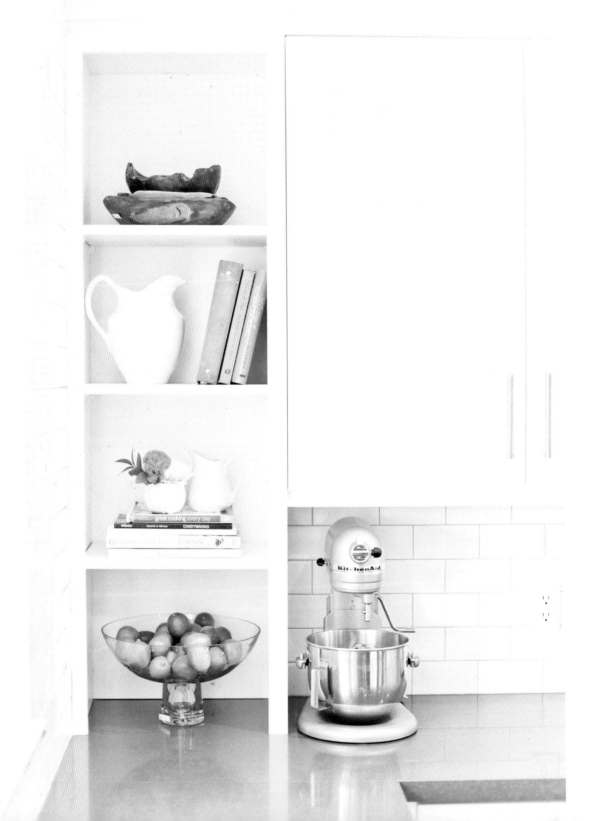

FANTASY ISLANDS

For Cami and Randon Jensen, creating a large and efficient enough kitchen in their existing home for their family of six (soon to be seven) presented quite a challenge. The Jensen's hired interior designer Pamela Jensen after several other designers had attempted—and failed—to produce a functional design worthy of the Jensen's large family and lifestyle.

In order to maximize the space, Pamela looked beyond the existing footprint of the kitchen and helped the homeowners add space from an adjacent, unused guest room. However, bringing the two rooms together as one created a new set of design challenges. The biggest problem was how to address the windows that now lined one entire wall of the new room. Pam's solution was to make the wall of windows a key design feature above the base cabinets. Because the size of the kitchen had increased substantially, the upper cabinets have never been missed.

The next order of business was to create multiple zones for cooking, eating, visiting, and working. Double islands, each with separate functions, are another highlight of the kitchen. The facade of each island base has a common and unique design element: chunky, mocha-stained legs supporting each corner.

To make the new kitchen feel cohesive, Pamela painted the cabinets and ceiling the same shade of white. A white subway tile backsplash, installed up to the ceiling, further completes the look. Grounding the entire space, a sultry porcelain tile designed to mimic limestone adds warmth while bringing in an element of nature.

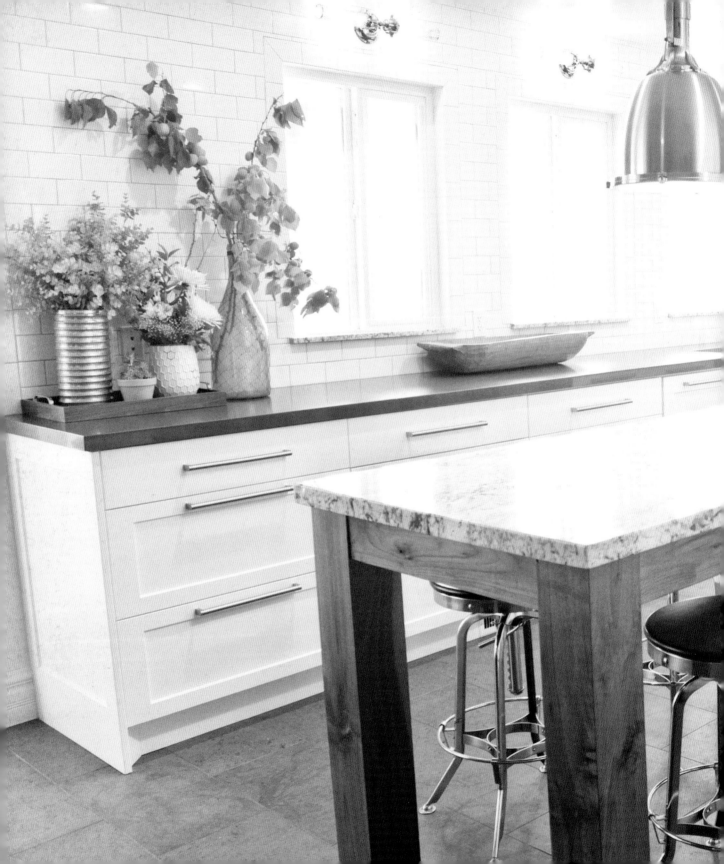

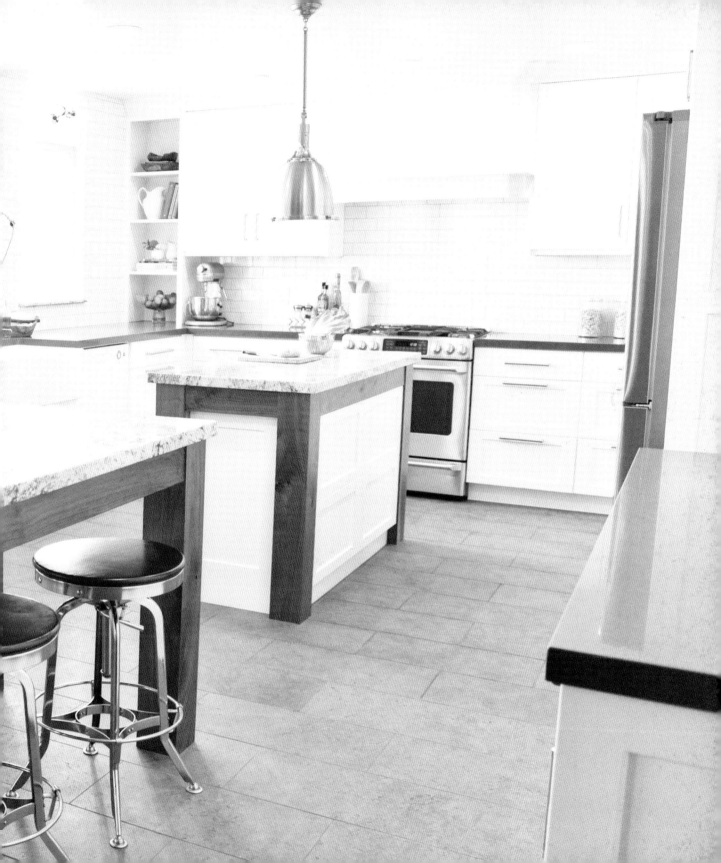

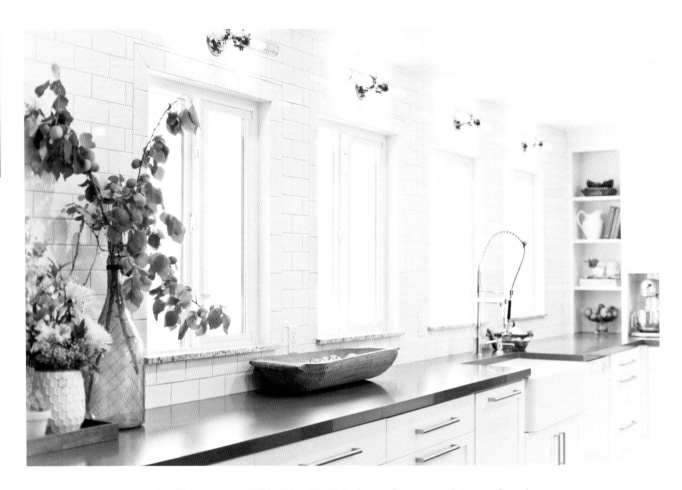

LONG WALLS OF WINDOWS, in lieu of upper cabinets, flood the kitchen with warm, natural light. The ample size of the kitchen provides plenty of storage in place of the uppers.

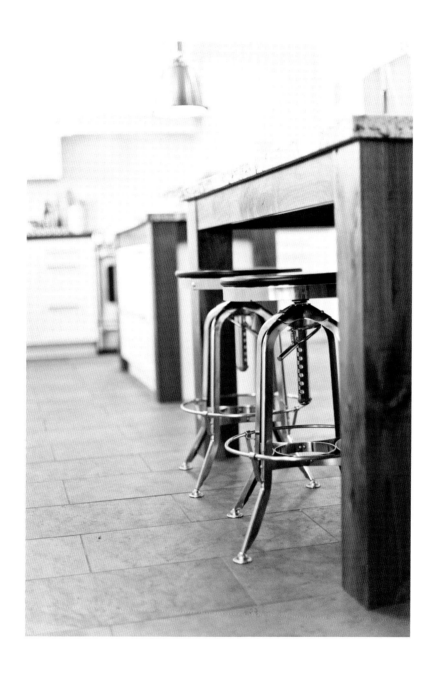

DOUBLE ISLANDS, similar yet contrasting in design, allow for cooking and prepping food in one zone while guests relax in another zone.

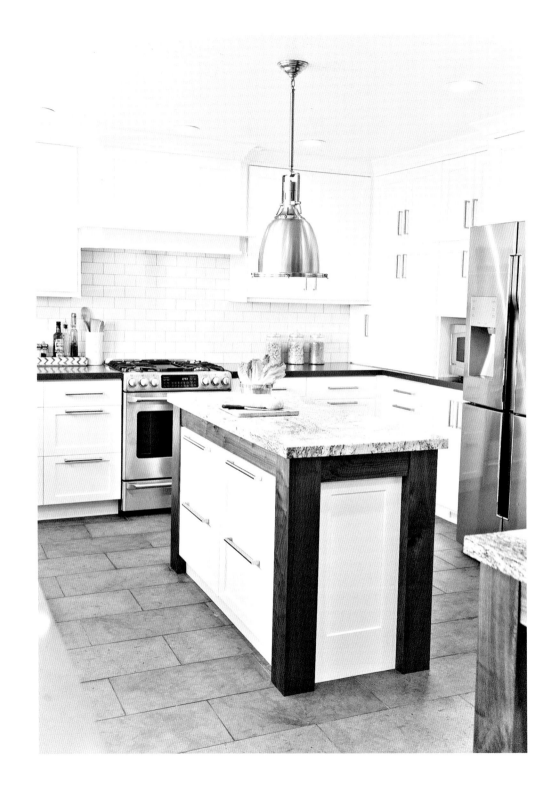

TYING IT TOGETHER

Elements of a Sanctuary

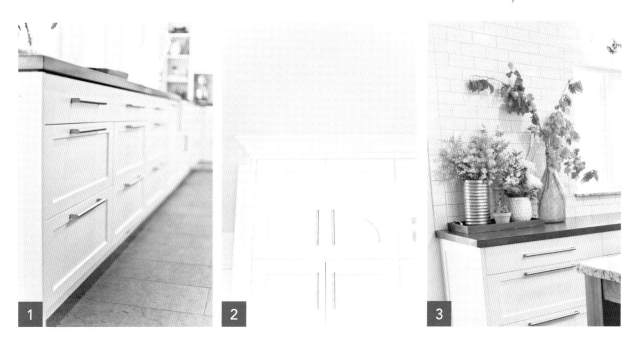

1 A LONG BANK of heavy-duty, deep drawers replace typical base cabinets, providing convenient access to multiple items. Double islands expand that space, offering even more, keeping the kitchen in *order*.

2 LOW-VOLTAGE LIGHT emanates from upper glass cabinets, drawing the eye up while simultaneously creating ambience.

3 CLIPPED BRANCHES and greenery add an element of *nature* to the space.

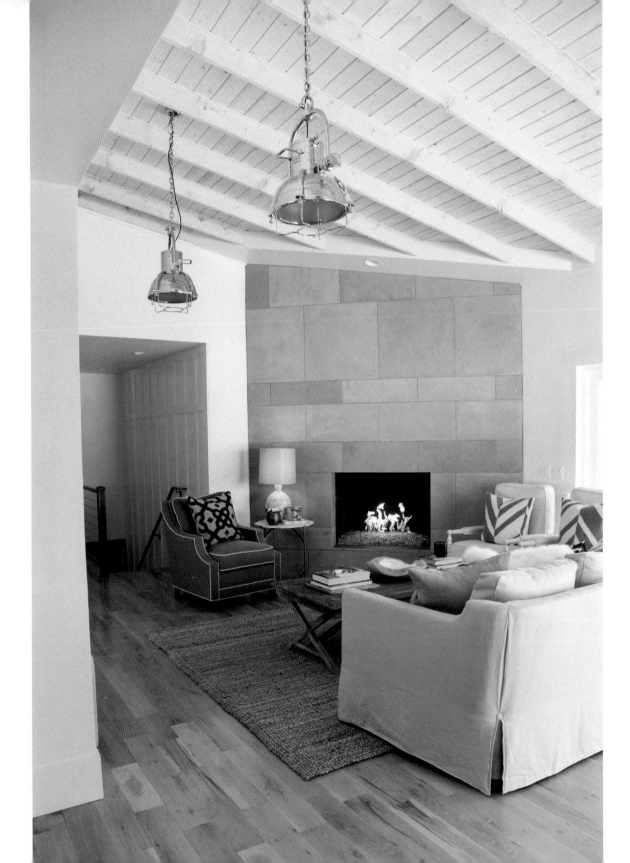

OLD HOUSE, NEW SPACE

Luckily for Jeff Olsen, when his wife, interior designer Tonya Olsen, first stepped into the 1960s rambler he had purchased while she was out of town, she saw the vision immediately. Despite the low ceilings, closed off spaces, awkward configuration and original decor, Tonya envisioned creating what she likes to refer to as a "modern industrial cottage."

With a need for space and plans for frequently hosting out-of-town friends and family, Jeff and Tonya tackled their biggest obstacle, limited square footage, head on. Rather than build out, they opened up the cavernous floor plan by tearing down walls and ripping out the existing eight-foot ceilings. Once the ceilings were gone, the Olsens were delighted by the architectural detail of the framing. The home was built using stick-frame construction, and the roof framing would add instant character and architectural appeal. As a result, the Olsens chose to leave the rafters exposed. The vaulted ceiling instantly created an expansive feeling in the space while projecting an impressive old-yet-new aesthetic.

The end result of the Olsens' renovations is an open floor plan full of character and style with plenty of gathering space.

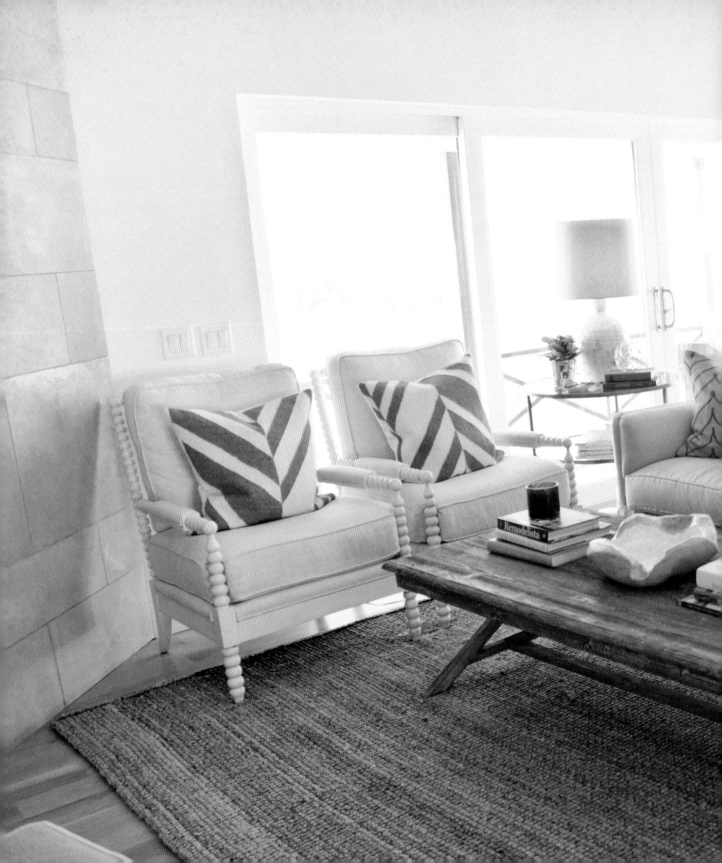

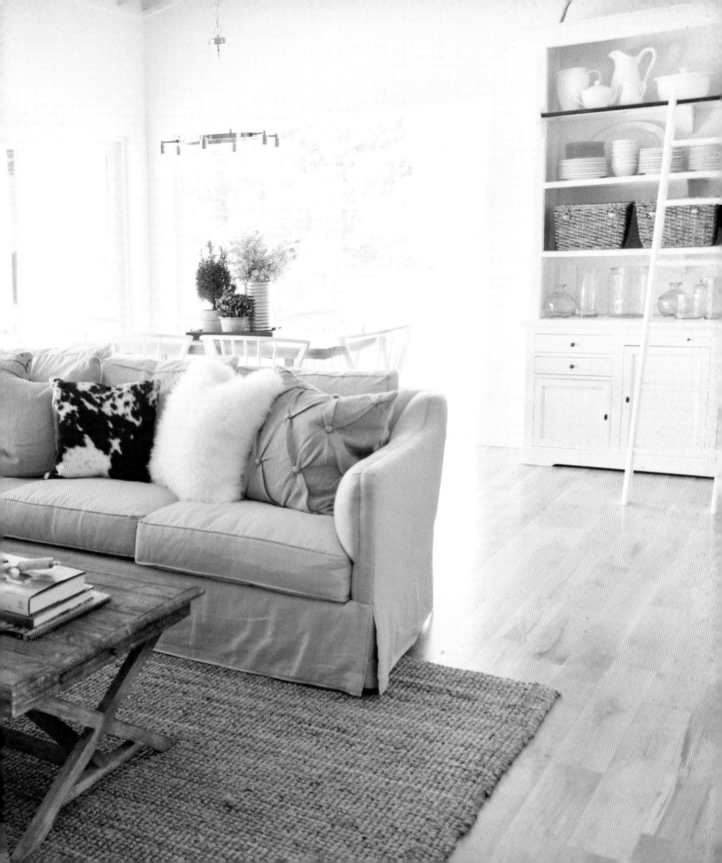

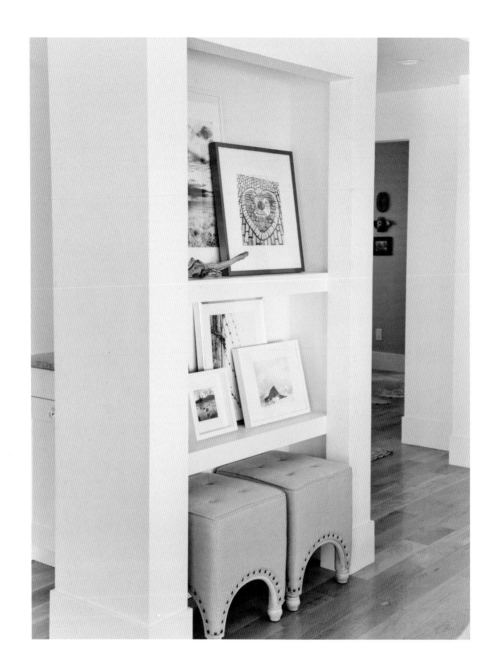

THIS CLEVER DESIGN adds a place to display treasures and store additional seating at the same time.

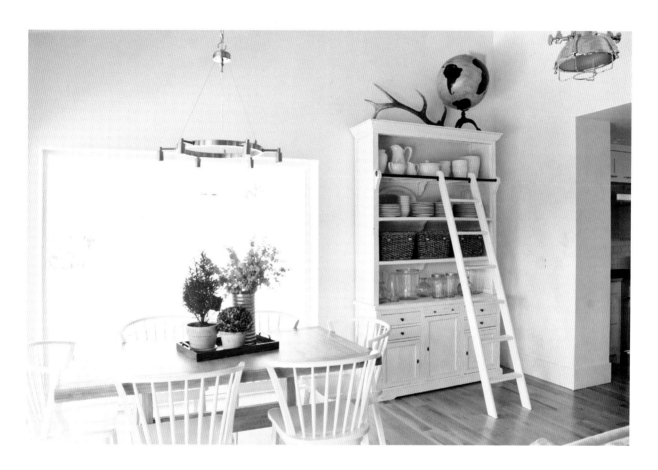

MODERN YET CLASSIC Windsor chairs provide ample seating for each member of the family. An open shelf hutch makes for easy access to serv-ingware, baskets full of linens, and various-sized glass jars used for flower arrangements when the Olsens entertain.

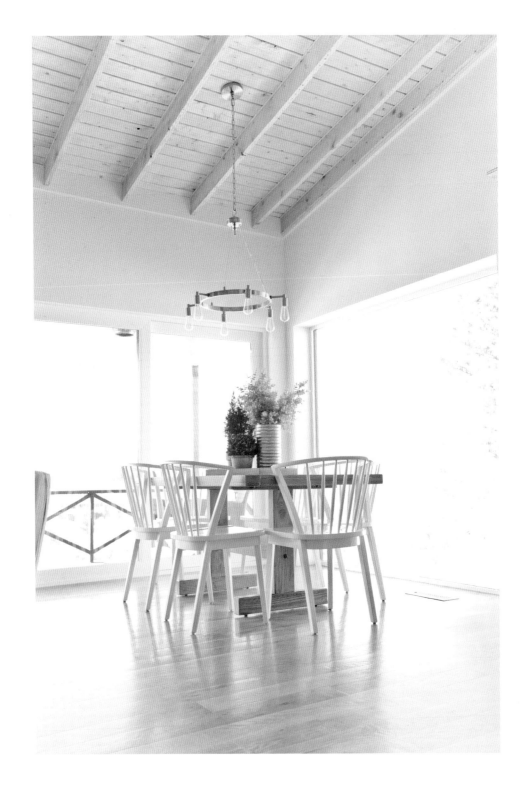

STRUCTURE

TYING IT TOGETHER

Elements of a Sanctuary

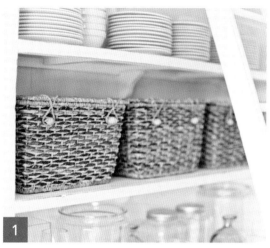
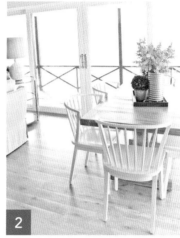
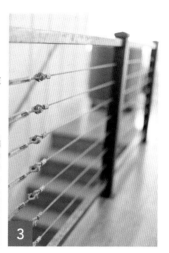

1 WICKER BASKETS add texture and dimension to the open hutch, while keeping linens and cutlery in *order*.

2 FLOOR-TO-CEILING WINDOWS flood the space with light while offering up an incredible view of *nature*.

3 A CUSTOM-DESIGNED decorative iron railing pulls in *details and materials* that complement the overall design of the space.

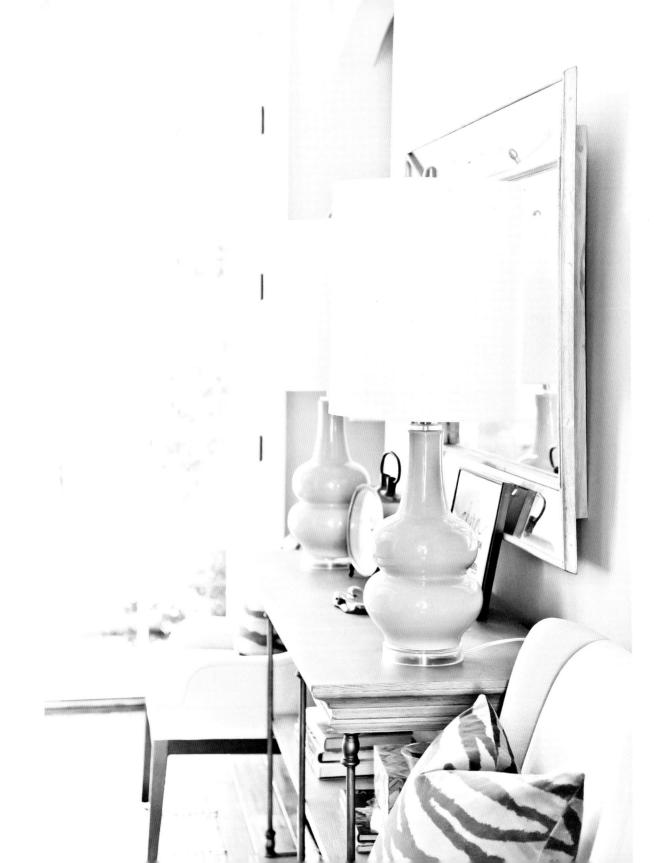

CROWD PLEASER

With four boys and a busy husband, it was no wonder that client Kristy Feller came into Liv Showroom seeking design help to create a functional gathering space for her family. Kristy needed a space that could not only hold up to wear and tear, but also serve as a place where the family could relax and enjoy time together. To keep up with a busy lifestyle, Kristy knew she needed a functional space that worked for all their desired activities.

The Feller home, nestled on a mountain edge with majestic views of the valley below, instinctively called for a softer color palette. Kristy knew she wanted a neutral background to allow for easy updates, such as swapping pillows and accessories for each holiday and season. The layout is perfect for family functions and gatherings. The kitchen, with a large island, adequately accommodates the family with additional seating in the adjoining breakfast and dining rooms. Designer Deboni Sacre worked with Kristy to create a dynamic atmosphere while maintaining harmony throughout the rest of the house. Practicality was at the root of every design decision.

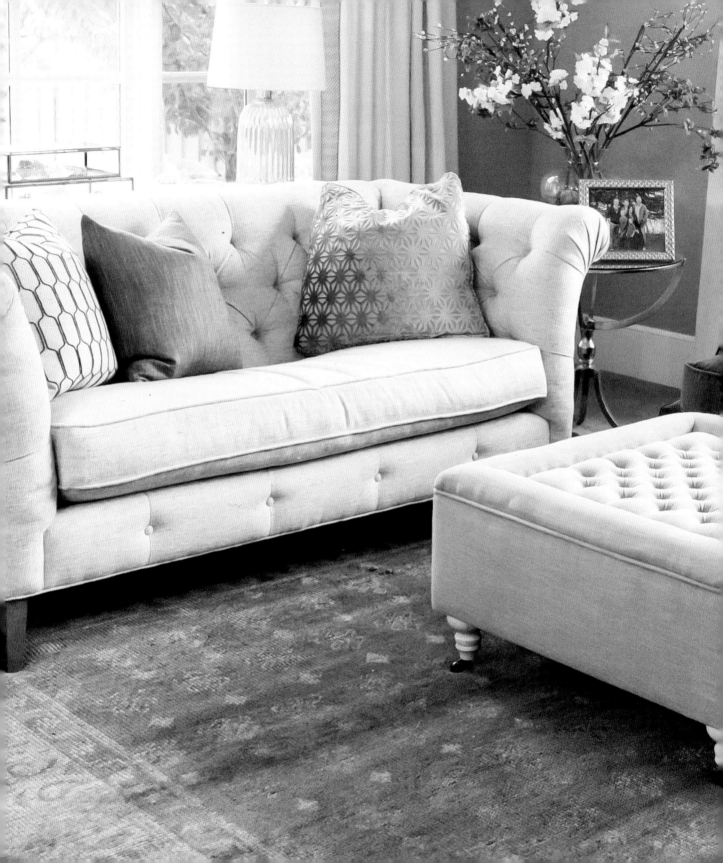

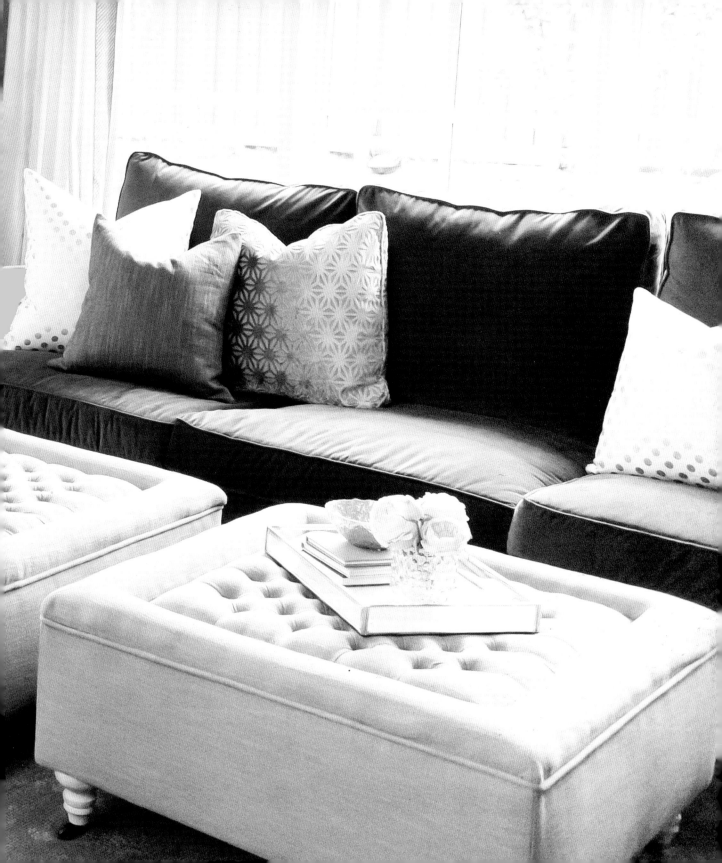

A SET OF CUSTOM-DESIGNED ottomans with casters serves double duty for leg propping and additional seating.

DECORATIVE YET PRACTICAL throw pillows can be used to adorn the oversized sofa or used by the children to sit on when family and friends gather in the space.

ADDING A SOFA-height console table behind the settee pulls it out into the space and creates a comfortable conversation area with the rest of the furniture. Tasteful lamps flank the multi-functional console table in addition to creatively displaying family treasures.

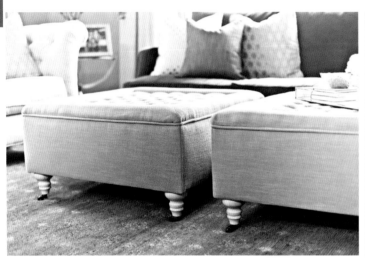

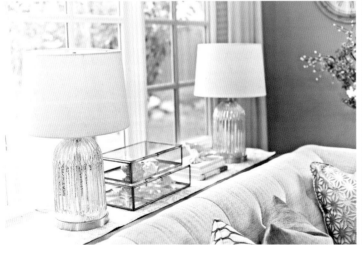

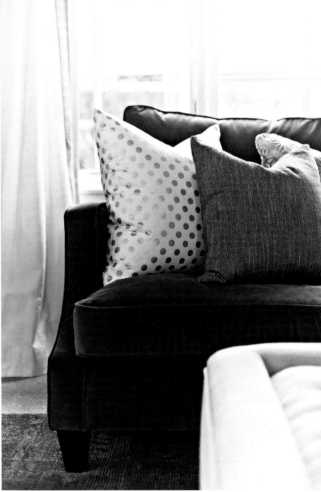

TYING IT TOGETHER

Elements of a Sanctuary

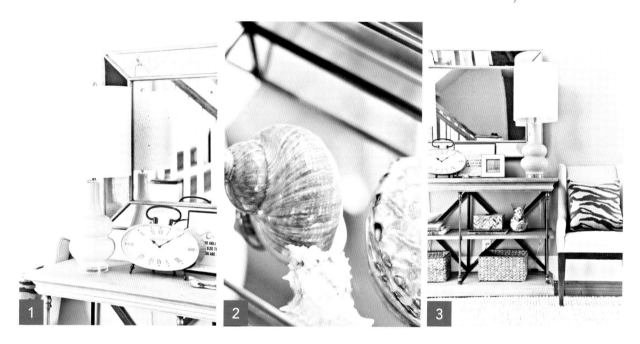

1   DECORATIVE LAMPS layered in front of an oversized mirror on the entry table add dimension and provide additional *light*.

2   THE FAMILY HAS A COLLECTION of seashells from their time spent on the East Coast. Reflective glass display boxes showcase *things that matter* and add a touch of nostalgia.

3   SEATING IN THE ENTRY provides an *in-between space* for guests to sit while removing their shoes.

Private and In-Between Spaces

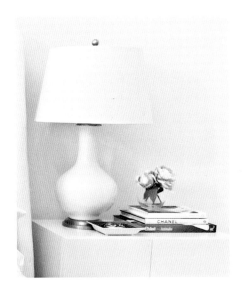

"My bedroom is my sanctuary. It's like a refuge."

—Vera Wang

PRIVATE AND IN-BETWEEN SPACES

Almost equal to the need for our connection to people is our need to connect with ourselves. Private spaces are created for physical and emotional rest and relaxation. Being alone can be a healthy, rejuvenating experience that allows us to reconnect with our own needs, goals, beliefs, values, and feelings. Private spaces can also help us create intimate one-on-one relationships with our spouses, children, or other loved ones. These relationships are essential to our emotional well-being.

Naturally, bedrooms can be deemed as private spaces, but consider other areas in a home that can double as both a private space and a gathering space depending on how they are engaged with the flow of the house. A small office can be a place for meeting but also for studying. A quaint living room can be used for an intimate talk with a child or a game with several friends.

An in-between space allows you to pull away from the core while still being a part of it at the same time. Areas such as niches, desks, window seats, alcoves, and even a simple corner can create an in-between space. These small areas create places to be "alone" but still be in the presence of the family and be socially connected. Many of our daily functions are private, but in our efforts to keep communal, our common areas must provide the ability to allow for those private functions within the larger functions of the room.

Private and in-between spaces allow time for pause and reflection. Life can be busy, stressful, and often overwhelming. For a home to properly support its household members, it should provide places of escape from the busyness of life.

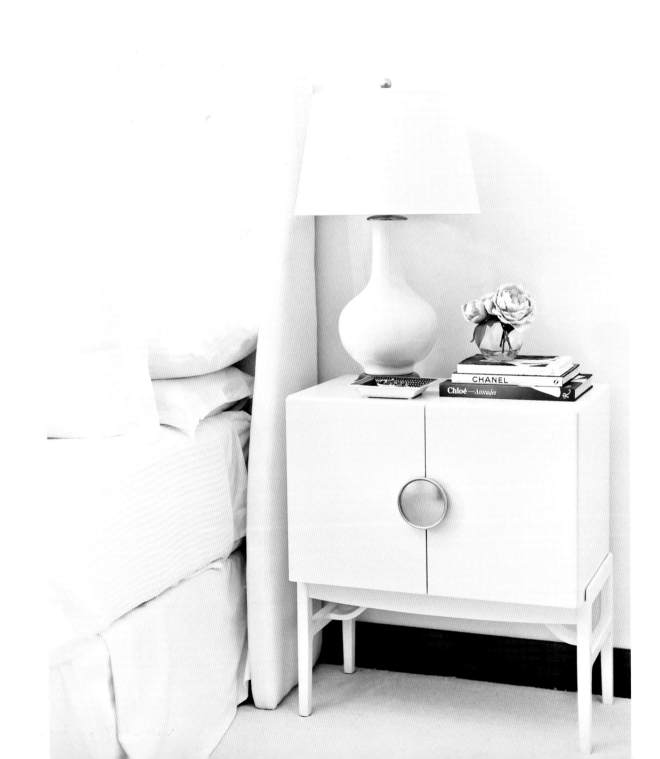

LIGHTEN UP

Some would say that a white-on-white color scheme is the opposite of warm and cozy, but Lisa Taggart disagrees. Her master bedroom, bathed in warm whites and creamy neutrals, is the epitome of a serene ethereal retreat. Lisa's objective was to keep the space crisp and clean and for it to serve as a private retreat for her and her husband from their hectic lifestyle. Lisa worked with interior designer Pamela Jensen to create this heavenly sanctuary.

A minimalistic design approach allows the space to feel uncluttered and distraction-free. Metallic accents like the burnished gold finish on the nightstand, lamp, and chandelier add a hint of elegance. Tufting adds subtle character to the upholstered headboard, which was designed to frame a sea of billowy white linens across the bed. The texture of a plush sheepskin rug grounds the bed to the space and connects it to a comfortable seating area. A supple leather club chair next to a warm and inviting fireplace is a bold yet complementary contrast to the rest of the space.

This luxurious retreat serves as the perfect place to get away.

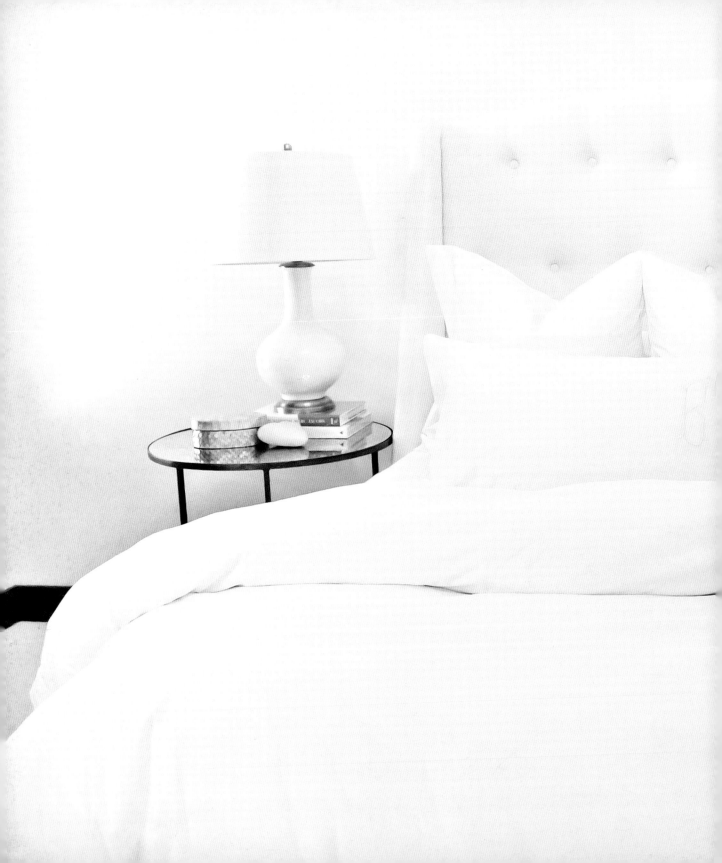

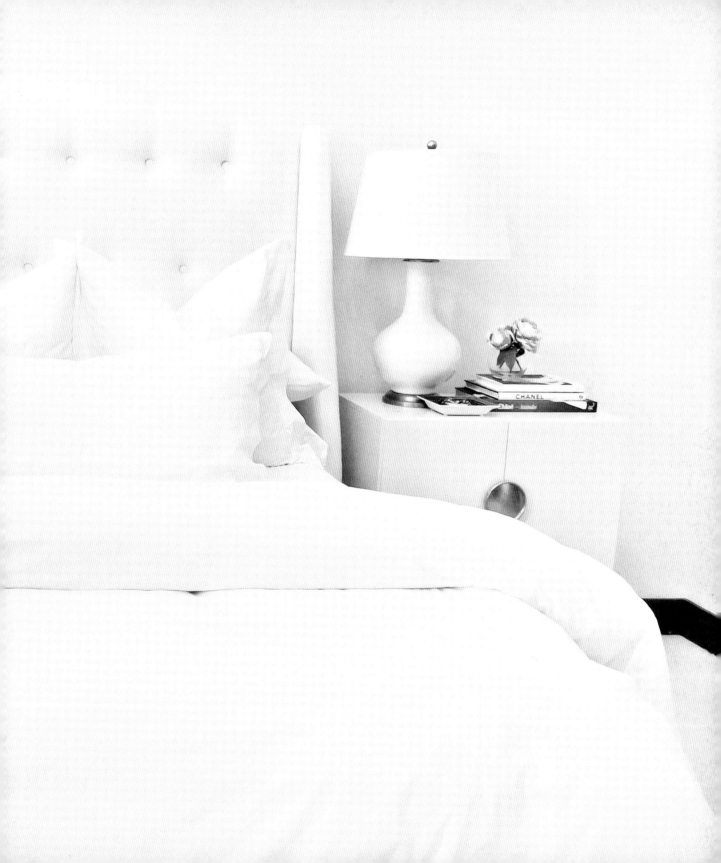

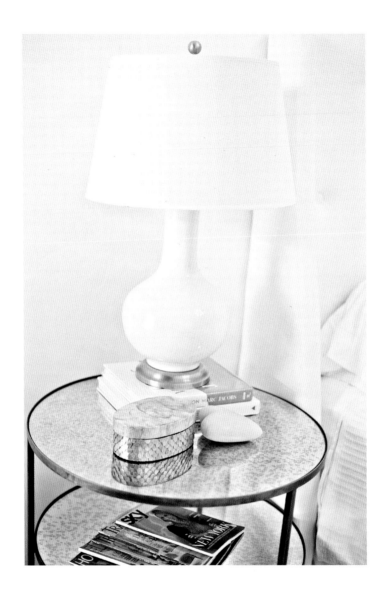

A MIRRORED SIDE TABLE, finished in antique gold, reflects a shimmery opulence into the room. Antiqued smokey glass adds a hint of understated glamour.

TYING IT TOGETHER

Elements of a Sanctuary

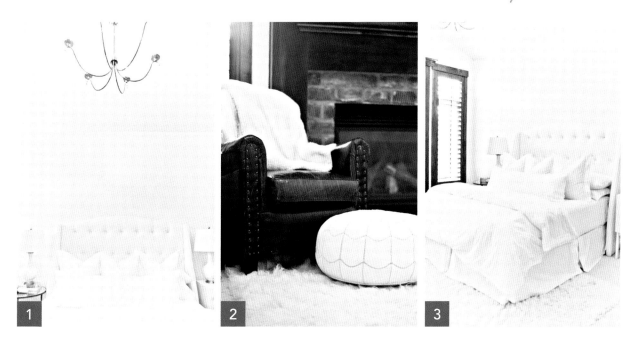

1 THE PLACEMENT and visual weight of the chandelier brings the lofty ceiling down to *human scale.*

2 A MASTER BEDROOM serves as a private retreat for *meditation* and *reflection.* A warm fire and a comfortable leather club chair paired with a leather pouf create the perfect place to read and relax.

3 SIMPLICITY AND ORDER go hand in hand with white linen bedding.

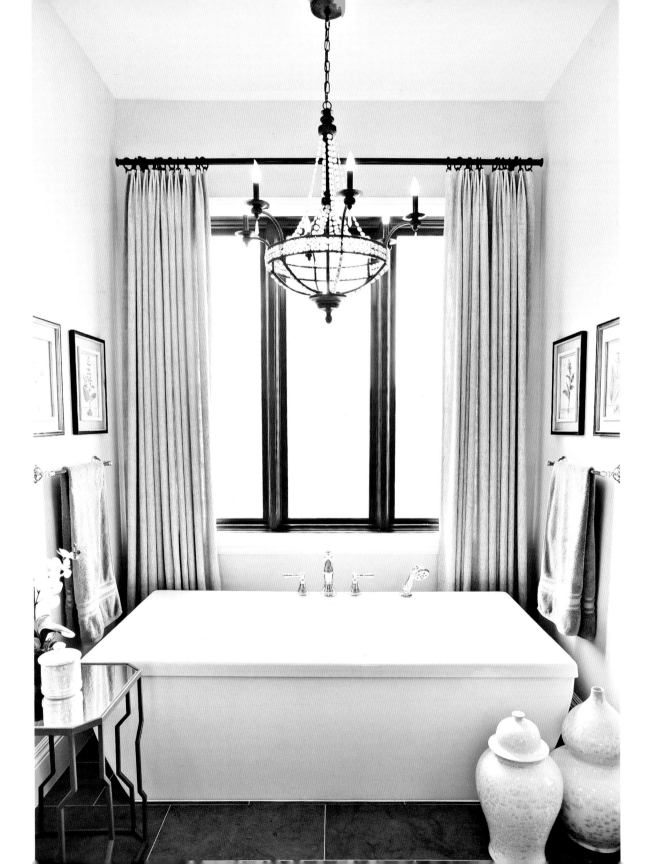

ESCAPE AT HOME

If you think you can't afford a luxurious, spa-like bathroom, think again. Interior designer Pamela Jensen pulled a few tricks out of her sleeve to create a blissful master bath retreat for Joyce and Brian Smith. Pam's secret? She knew exactly where to spend the money . . . and where to save it.

The biggest cost saver was installing porcelain tile with the look and feel of natural limestone. The stain-, scratch-, and moisture-resistant surface adds a down-to-earth look without the maintenance of natural stone. Money is better spent in finishing touches like the marble mosaic floor tile in the shower.

In a room full of hard surfaces, drapery panels soften the surroundings and frame the large-scale picture window. The Smiths close the panels for optimum opacity and light a few candles to further create the spa-like experience. A glamorous chandelier creates a focal point above the freestanding soaking tub.

We can't forget about location. A true getaway is typically located far from reality. While working with their architect, the Smith's consciously designed their master bath to be nestled away from the busy heart of the home.

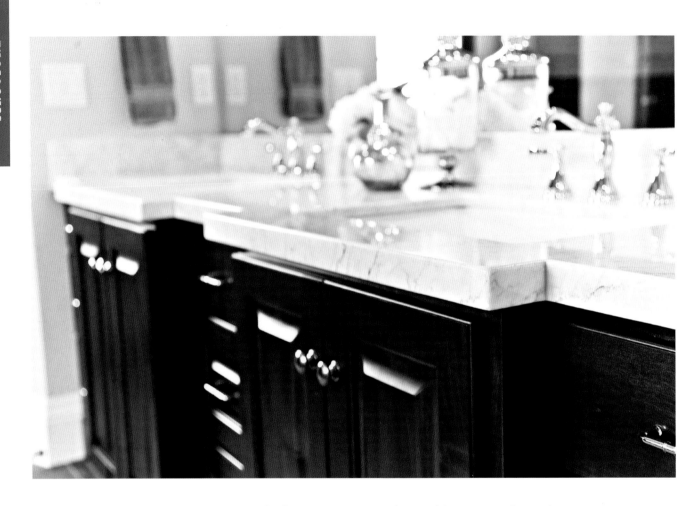

MARBLE COUNTERTOPS sit atop warm walnut cabinets, creating a time-less juxtaposition of finishes. Wall-to-wall mirrors expand the visual size of the space.

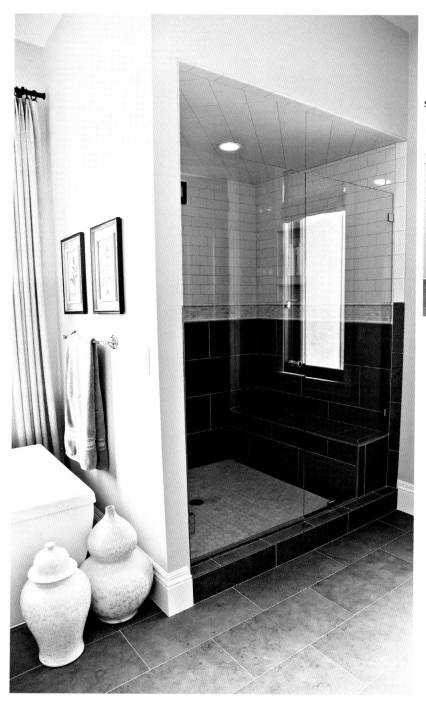

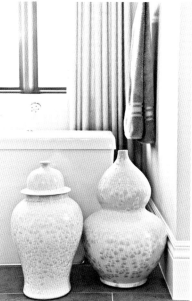

SOFT TONES and a simple design make this private place more relaxing. A frameless, European shower door keeps the space open and airy.

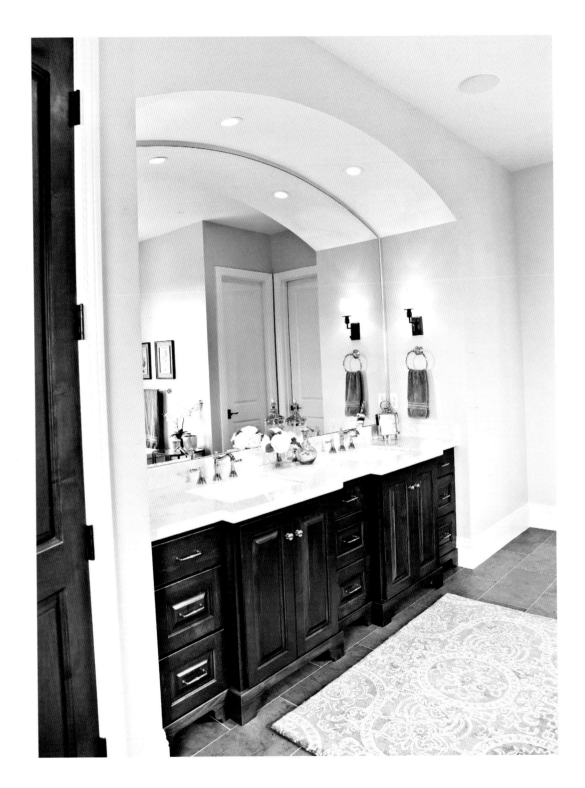

TYING IT TOGETHER

Elements of a Sanctuary

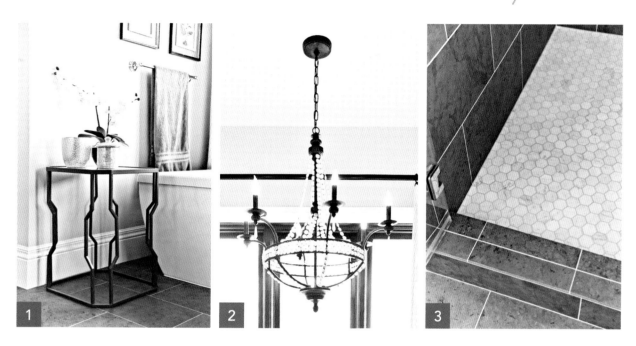

1 PLACING A SMALL TABLE next to the tub provides a prop to hold a good book and a little candlelight to further enhance the experience for *inspiration* and *meditation*.

2 THE SUBTLE LIGHT of a grand chandelier adds an elegant and stunning glow.

3 PORCELAIN FLOOR TILE combined with marble mosaic on the shower floor is a practical mix of *details and materials*.

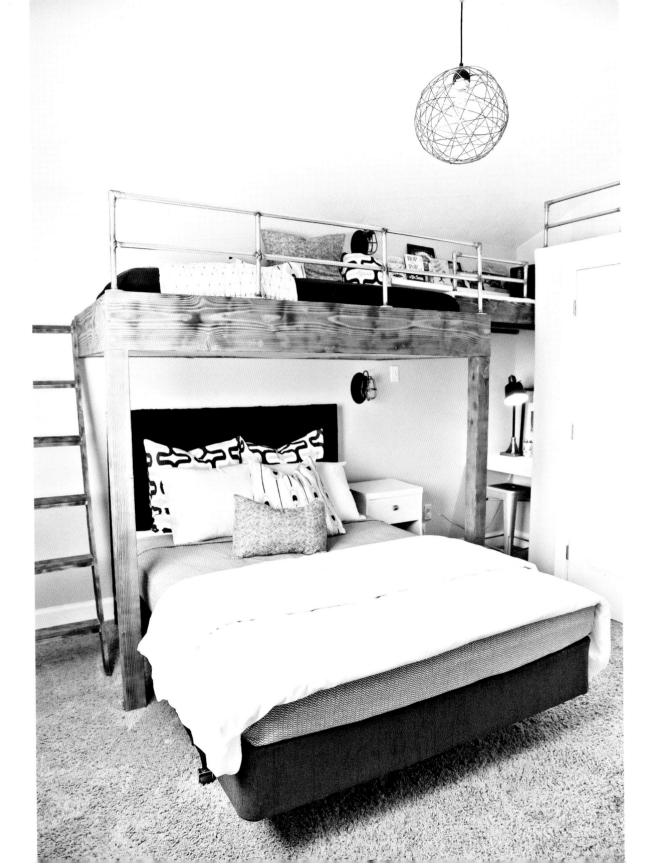

KIDDING AROUND

Designer Deboni Sacre had an interesting area in her boys' room to contend with. Above the boys' closet was a pocket of dead space that Deboni was sure could be transformed into something useful. The years she spent rocking her boys to sleep in their bedroom gave her plenty of time to gain inspiration. She finally decided to create a fun "getaway" once her boys were old enough. Deboni also wanted to design the space with built-in beds that would allow the bedroom to work for overnight guests if needed.

Deboni put her husband, Russell, to work tearing down the wall, building the beds, and adding a fun shelving unit. In exchange for Russell's hard work, he offered to hang pictures of his new Camaro or "Daddy's fast car" as three-year-old Cooper calls it. The room is a special getaway and allows for little spots all around the room for Elliott and Cooper to have their own space.

Deboni let the boys select the color scheme and fabrics for the room while providing a little direction. Together they decided to surround the room in the things the boys' love . . . all things fast: dirt bikes, race cars, airplanes.

A CORNER DESK in this playful kids' room allows privacy for a myriad of functions, including homework, drawing, or building with the boys' favorite toys.

EMPTY SPACE above the closet was uncovered to create a fun private loft space for playing, reading, or simply getting away. A pulley system adds a fun element and makes the space functional.

THE QUEEN BED is plenty big for a three-year-old, but serves double duty as a guest bed.

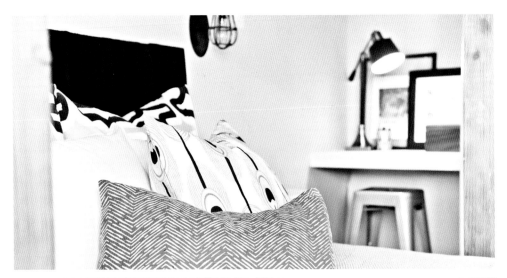

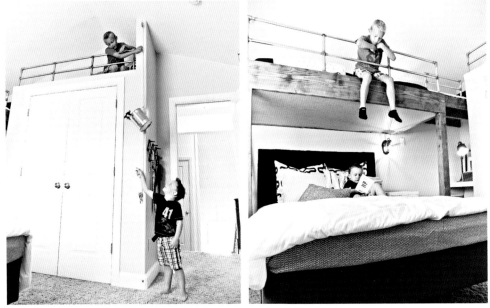

TYING IT TOGETHER
Elements of a Sanctuary

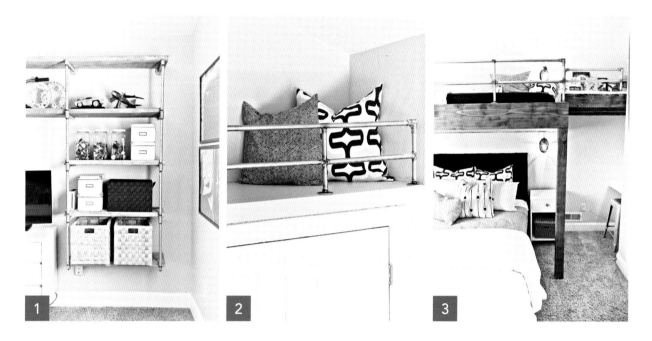

1   THE SHELVES DOUBLE as displays for the *things that matter*. For these boys, that includes anything that goes fast.

2   A TUCKED-AWAY *private space* doubles as a perfect place for *meditation* and *reflection*.

3   SCONCES WERE ADDED next to both beds as reading lights to create a variety of *lighting* for moods and tasks. A desk lamp adds more variety.

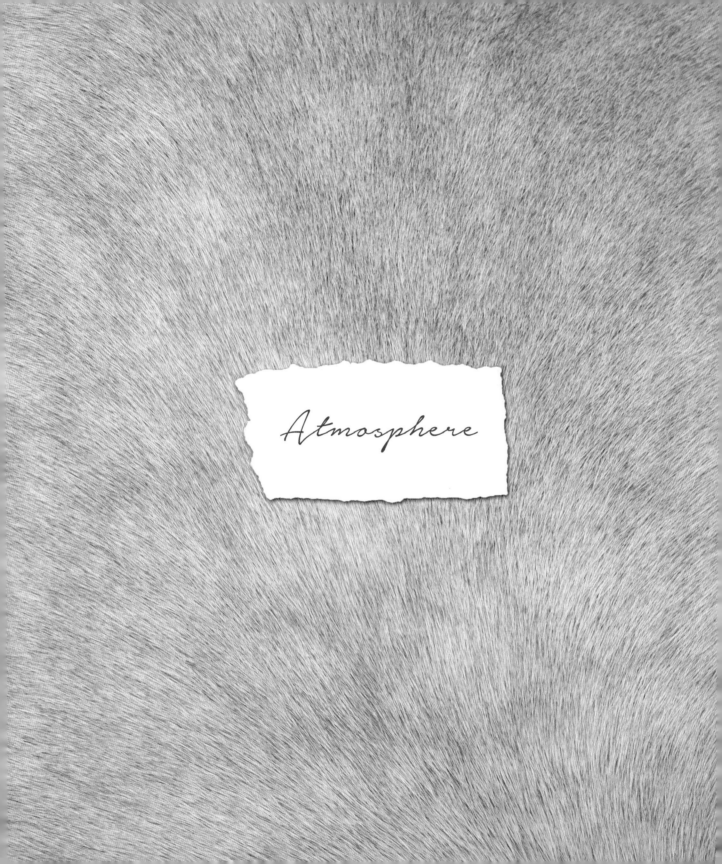

Atmosphere

ATMOSPHERE

A sanctuary is about surrounding yourself with things that make you feel good and enhancing your experience in a space. It's not about keeping up with the Joneses; it's about nurturing your soul.

Atmosphere follows the structure of a home. If the elements of the structure are limited, an enhanced atmosphere can balance the mental, emotional, and spiritual attributes of a space. A poorly designed atmosphere can only add to the disorder of an inadequately designed structure.

In designing our spaces, we create a variety of "tones" or moods. Some of these moods are sophisticated or lively, cozy or casual. The best spaces offer diversity in desired experiences and moods for the activities of a space. Architect and author of *Creating the Inspired House*, John Connell, says it best: "The ineffable quality of a well-designed space goes beyond what we can see with our eyes." Sound, touch, and smell also directly affect our atmosphere.

A relaxing mood is set with soothing colors, dim accent lighting, soft textures, and relaxing sounds. An excitable atmosphere is easy to create with intense colors, contrast, and bright lighting.

Our mental state is the element of our personal wellness that is most influenced and affected by atmosphere. An atmosphere can easily uplift a mood and just as effortlessly create a mood of discomfort. The elements combined to create the space drive this response. One important aspect of a person's overall mental well-being is directly related to the environment they are in.

Interior Reflection

ASK YOURSELF THE FOLLOWING QUESTIONS WHEN CONTEMPLATING
THE **MENTAL ATMOSPHERE** OF YOUR HOME:

1. How can my home support the mental health I want for myself and for my family?
2. Am I sensitive to light, color, or sound?
3. Do I prefer an ample amount of natural light or a dimly-lit interior?
4. How does color affect my mental health? Do I prefer bright, soothing, warm, or cool colors?
5. How does sound affect the atmosphere in my home? Is my family typically loud or quiet? Do the objects in my home thrill my senses?

Light and Sound

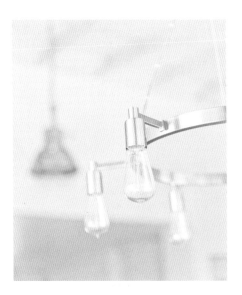

"Light is the magical ingredient that
makes or breaks a space."

—Benjamin Noriega-Ortiz

LIGHT AND SOUND

It is well known that environments filled with sufficient natural light can improve health, relieve depression, and aid in sleep habits. Light is more than sight. It creates warmth in our souls and enhances our experiences. The contrast of light and shadows can lead us around a space.

You need a variety of lighting, both natural and artificial. Combining outside light with inside light plays an important role in creating a balanced atmosphere. Max Jacobson, Murray Silverstein, and Barbara Winslow, authors of *Patterns of Home: The Ten Essentials of Enduring Design* point out that we are comfort loving creatures. We turn toward the sun, seeking light and warmth because we need sunlight to nourish both spirit and body.

The optimum formula for lighting a room is to have natural light coming in on two sides. Jacobson, Silverstein, and Winslow point out that "interior light quality is influenced by the size, style, and location of the windows and doors." Strategize the placement of these openings to let in nature and light. In addition, light can be softened by using window treatments and shades. Use shading devices to control the light and temperature.

The more options for lighting, the better. Rooms should have various ways to be lit. Artificial light allows you to create moods for a variety of activities during certain times of day. Artificial light creates zones for activities such as reading or working. Use dimmers whenever possible for your artificial lighting. It allows flexibility for the moods you want and the activities you need performed in a space. Mirrored furniture and framed mirrors reflect light and space—use them to your advantage in a small room.

Sound isn't necessarily an element of design, but it is a part of creating atmosphere. Music and sounds add to or detract from the visual atmosphere you create.

Sound doesn't just mean music. Keep in mind the effect that the sounds from outside will have on the atmosphere. You'll also want to consider controlling the sounds of an active home (such as footsteps, loud conversation, or sound that carries from televisions, computers, and musical instruments).

Adding textiles such as window treatments and rugs can help absorb sounds and keep loud sounds from destroying a created atmosphere. In planning your space, consider how you want music to be a part of your home. Music can be brought in to enliven or to relax or to create any mood in between.

Many people have music rooms. To be effective, these rooms should not only have instruments, but ample comfortable seating and a nice atmosphere to draw people in to use the space. A small living room can double as a living room and music room.

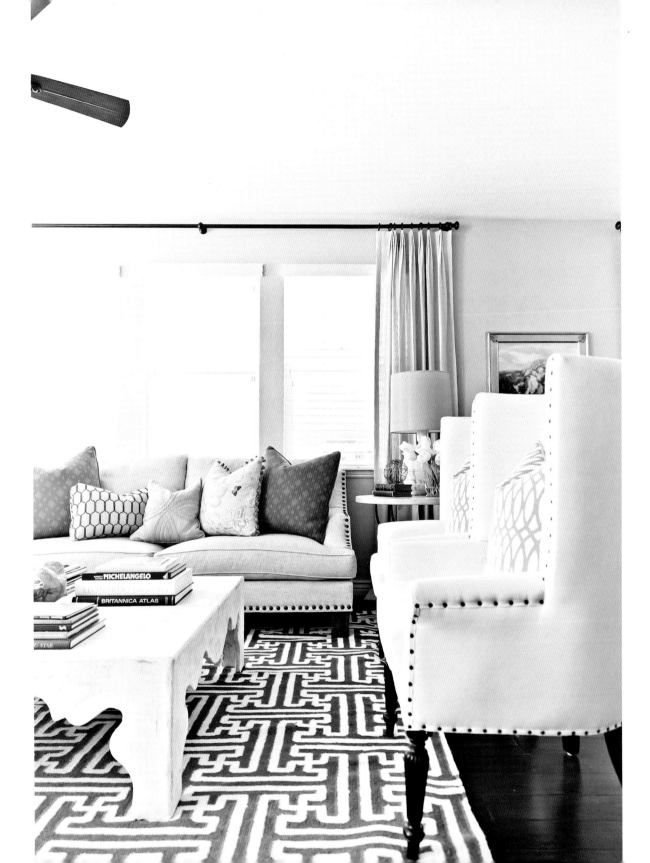

ALL IN THE FAMILY

Christy Petrie's family spends more time at home than most since she home-schools her four children. She realized how important her environment was for her family and sought help from designer Pamela Jensen to turn her family room into a gathering place. The main requests were to have as much seating as possible for large extended-family gatherings and to make the space bright and airy.

The home they purchased was formerly a builder's model, so the interior was designed to be neutral. While they loved the home overall, the dark wood floors, tan walls, and dark cabinetry didn't reflect their personal taste. They wanted a bright and airy space with a lot of white and cream with pops of color throughout.

Pamela got to work brightening the space with light and color. To illuminate the drab color scheme, she selected a soft yet warm gray for the walls, multiple tones of white and cream in the furniture and decor, and white finish work. Additional accent lighting was added with a table lamp and two floor lamps.

Pamela tackled the seating challenge full force by adding fourteen seats to the existing dining area, including built-in benches, a comfortable and oversized sofa, two high-back chairs, a stool, two bright poufs, and a love seat. An area rug in a bold color anchored the seating group, and bursts of colorful pillows were scattered throughout the arrangement.

Originally, the fireplace had a small mantel that felt out of proportion to the overall space. Pamela beefed up the look by adding a larger one and taking it all the way to ceiling. The dramatic effect adds additional white detailing while creating a stronger focal point. On one wall is a gallery of photos of extended family and a collection of the family's favorite books.

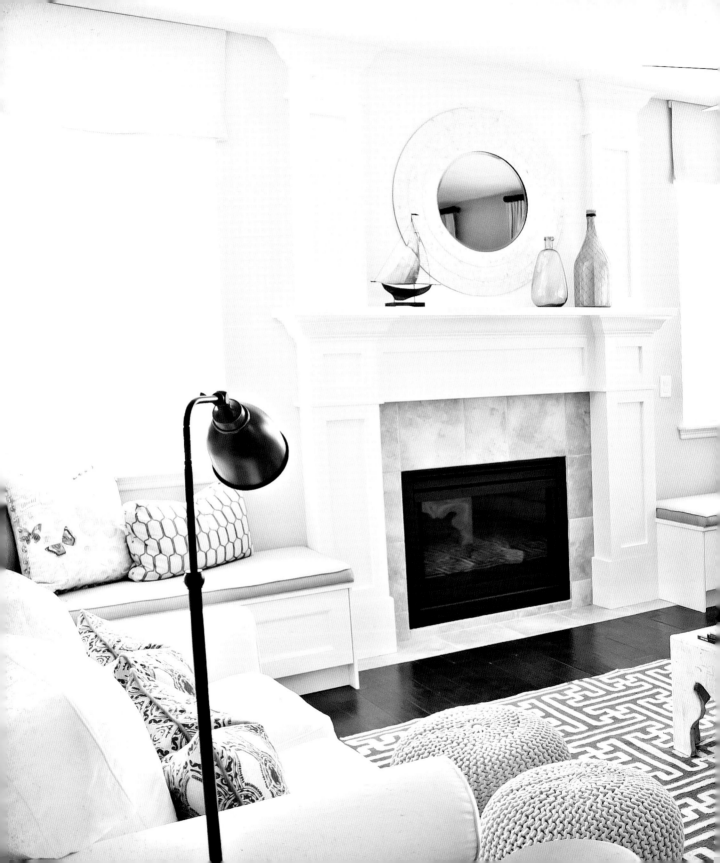

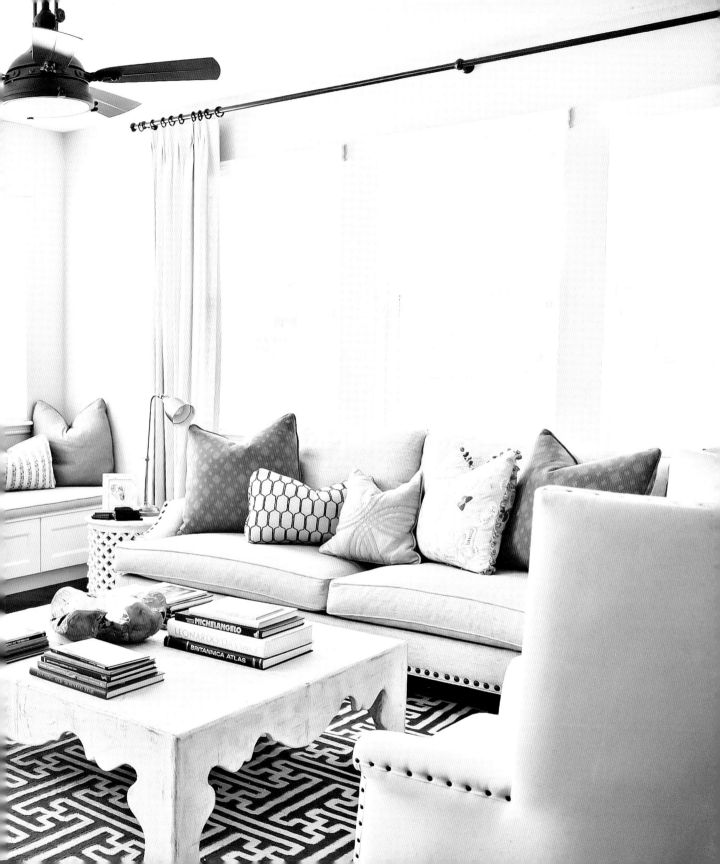

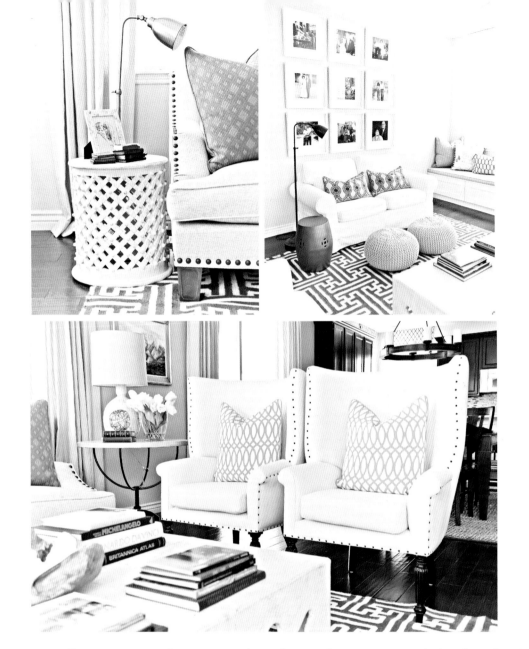

A TASK LAMP illuminates a reading area on the sofa. Window treatments behind can be drawn to control the natural light and temperature.

NATURAL LIGHT from the window above the bench bathes the space with sun. Additional accent lighting allows for family members to be doing various activities around the room.

LARGE-SCALE CHAIRS allow some separation between the rooms and add a great design feature as well.

TYING IT TOGETHER

Elements of a Sanctuary

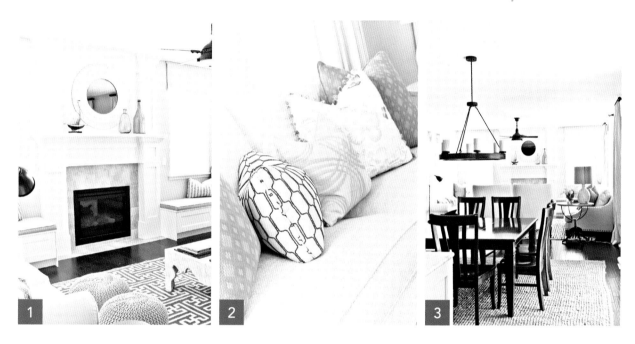

1   **STORAGE BENCHES** flank the fireplace and keep blankets and additional pillows in *order*.

2   **A VARIETY OF COLOR** in throw pillows and the area rug enlivens the space.

3   **SEATING FOR UP TO TWENTY-FIVE** is scattered throughout three rooms, creating an abundant *gathering space* for large groups.

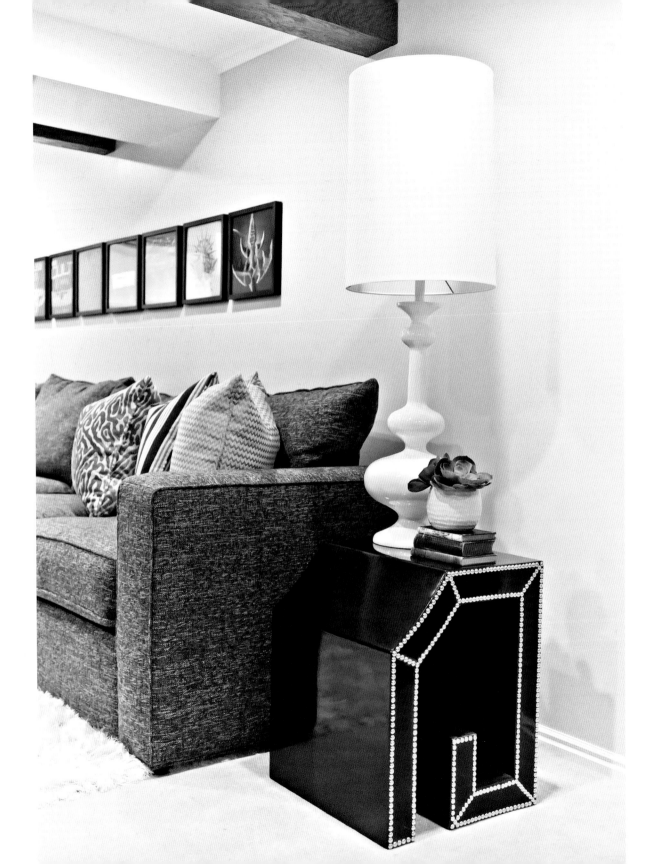

FROM BLEAK TO BRILLIANT

Kassi Capener has been a client of Pamela Jensen for some time. Together they've worked on designing the family's dental practice office and on various rooms in her home over the years. Instead of building a new home, the couple decided to buy an existing home on a large lot in an established neighborhood, surrounded by full-grown trees and mature landscaping. The choice was a good one, because the element of nature makes this home a true sanctuary.

The duo's latest project involved turning a dark 1970s basement with unsightly window wells into a place for the family to gather and enjoy spending time. Kassi wanted the space to be informal and used as a playroom, with plenty of seating for casual entertaining and watching movies.

The biggest challenge was how to design within the long, narrow footprint of the room. Having a space for a large TV was important to her husband, Randy, and being able to hide the TV was important to Kassi. Pam's solution was to design wall-to-wall built-ins with sliding barn doors on both sides of the fireplace. With a slide of the door, the television is hidden and storage shelves are revealed.

Since the basement has low ceilings, it seems the obvious choice would have been to paint the cabinets white. However, Pamela chose to paint them a dark charcoal to create depth and give the room a lounge feel. The exposed brick on the fireplace was updated with a gravel-gray paint to create contrast next to the cabinets.

Pamela installed roller shades a few inches bigger than the actual window size to create the illusion of length. The semi-transparent shades hide the garish window wells and still allow light into the space.

The result is a beautiful and functional basement for the whole family to enjoy.

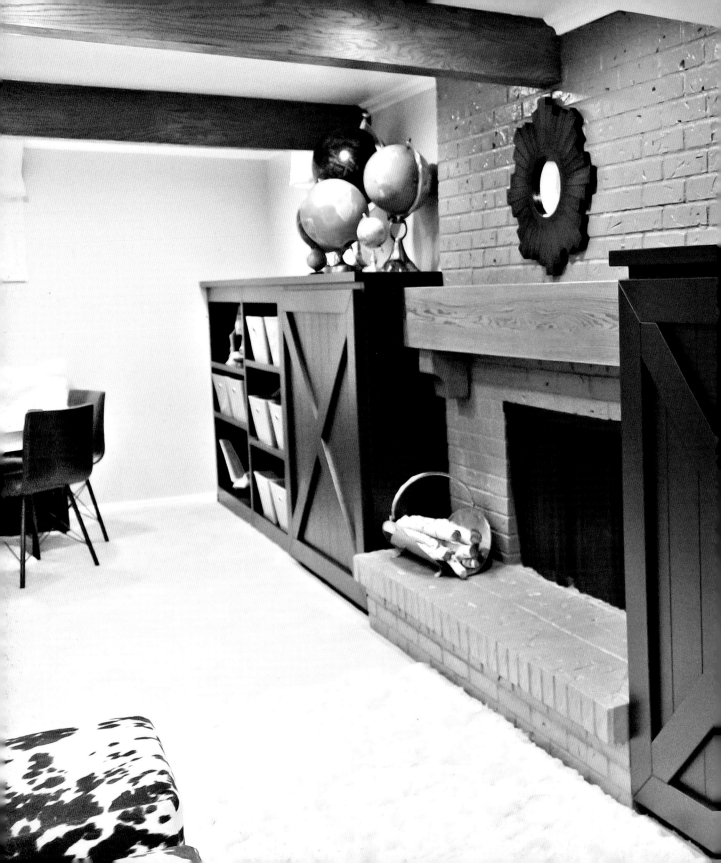

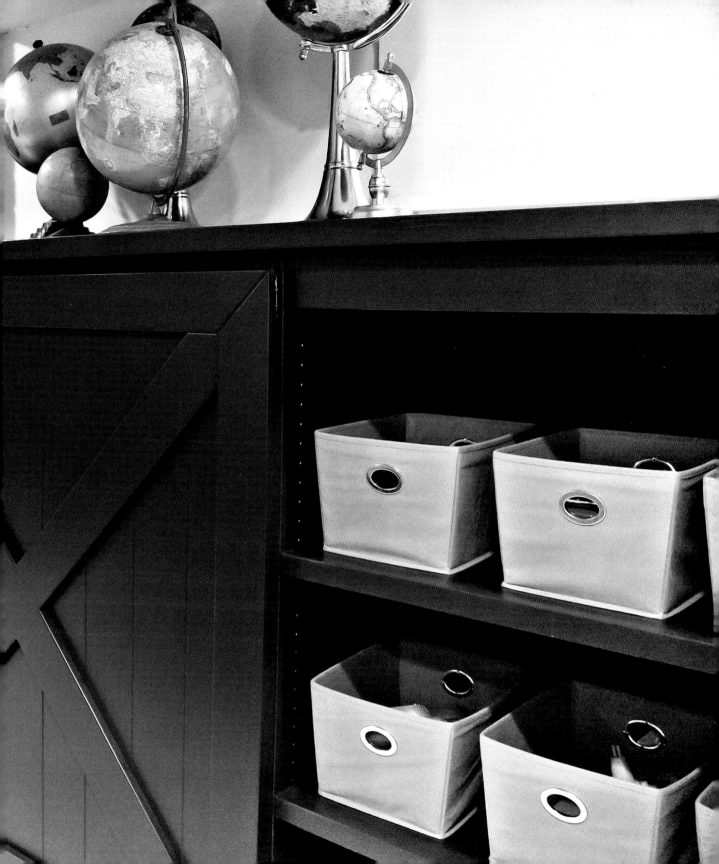

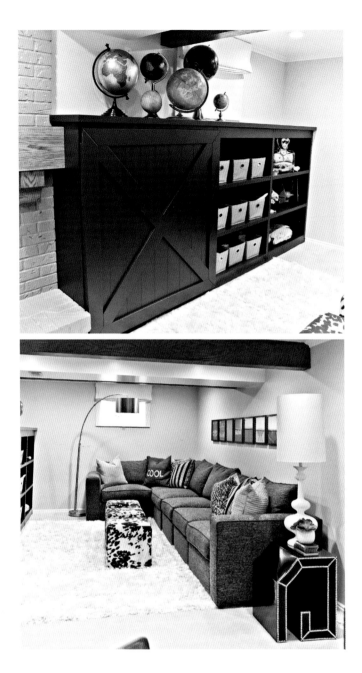

THIS CLEVER CABINET design accommodates a large television and shelves for storage. The sliding barn doors expose one or the other.

ADDITIONAL LIGHTING IS KEY to a small basement space. Recessed lights were installed in the ceiling, while a floor and table lamp provide accent lighting.

TYING IT TOGETHER
Elements of a Sanctuary

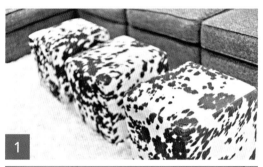

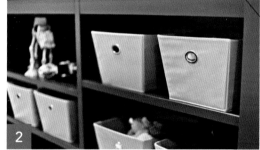

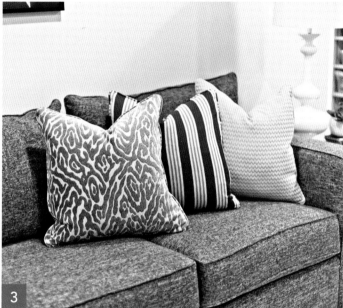

1   CUBES COVERED IN COWHIDE fabric double as seating, making this room the perfect *gathering space* for a large party.

2   BUILT-INS fill up one wall, creating lots of opportunities for storage. Fabric bins keep toys, games, and miscellaneous items in *order*.

3   A FUN COLOR SCHEME of gray, white, navy, and yellow keep the room inviting and give it *personality*.

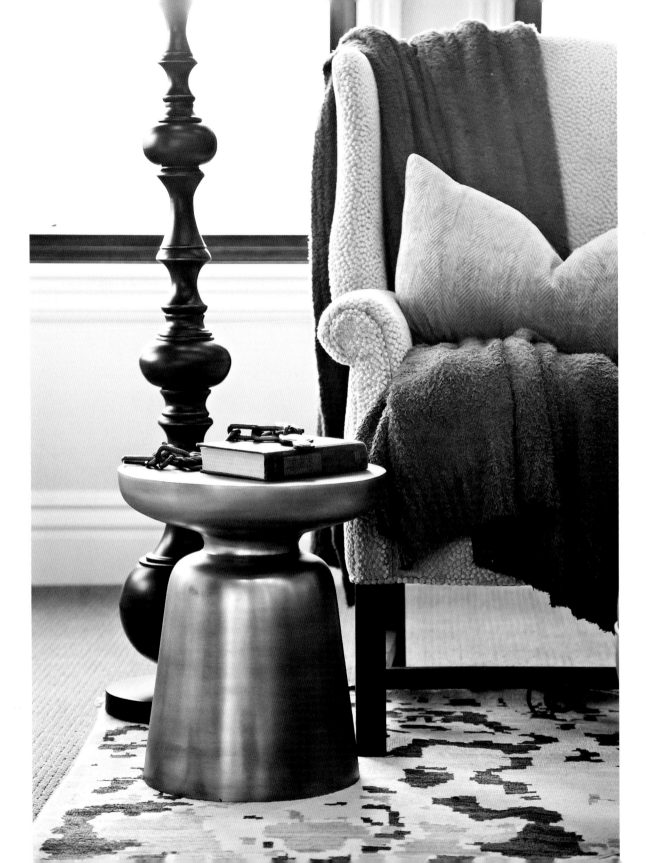

LOFTY APPROACH

Vaulted ceilings can make a room feel spacious, but sometimes that spaciousness can overwhelm. Designer Pamela Jensen incorporated a little-known design secret to help make the cavernous space of Rachelle Olsen's great room feel more inviting. She "layered" light by adding table and floor lamps to the seating area, drawing the eye down and making the space feel more intimate and cozy. Combined with a trio of oversized windows with transoms, the Olsens' great room is flooded with an ample amount of ambient, task, and natural light.

Light bounces off the multidimensional tongue-and-groove ceiling, which was finished with a semigloss paint. Contrasting that, the smooth textured walls painted with a satin finish prevent a harsh reflection from the multitude of light sources.

To further give the space a light yet sophisticated feeling, Pamela introduced a tone-on-tone color palette including soft neutrals in the furniture and finishes. An extra-long sofa, paired with a set of classic wing-back chairs and a tufted leather ottoman creates a comfortable conversation area. The overall effect suits the Olsens' style perfectly.

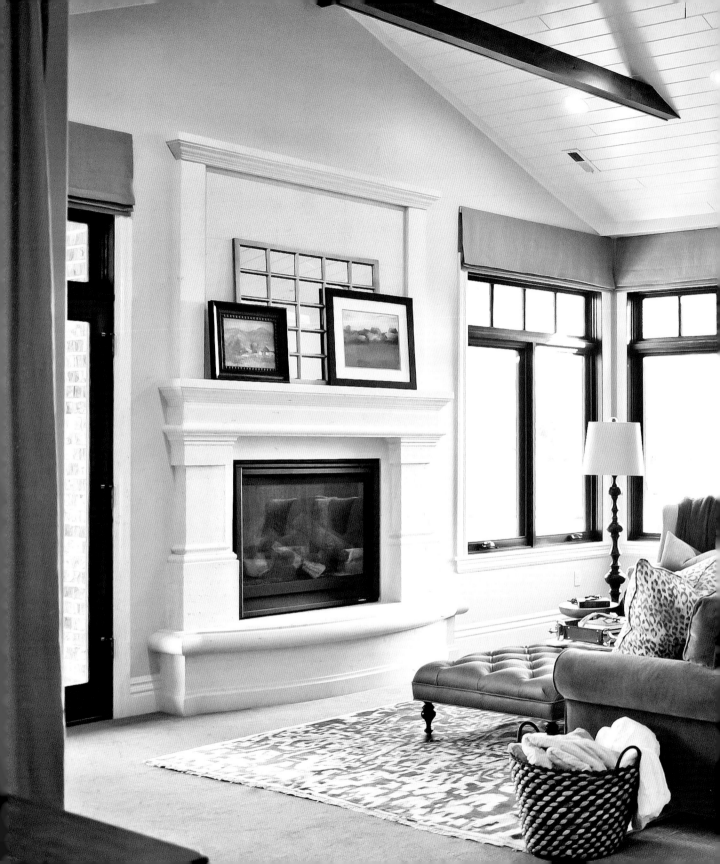

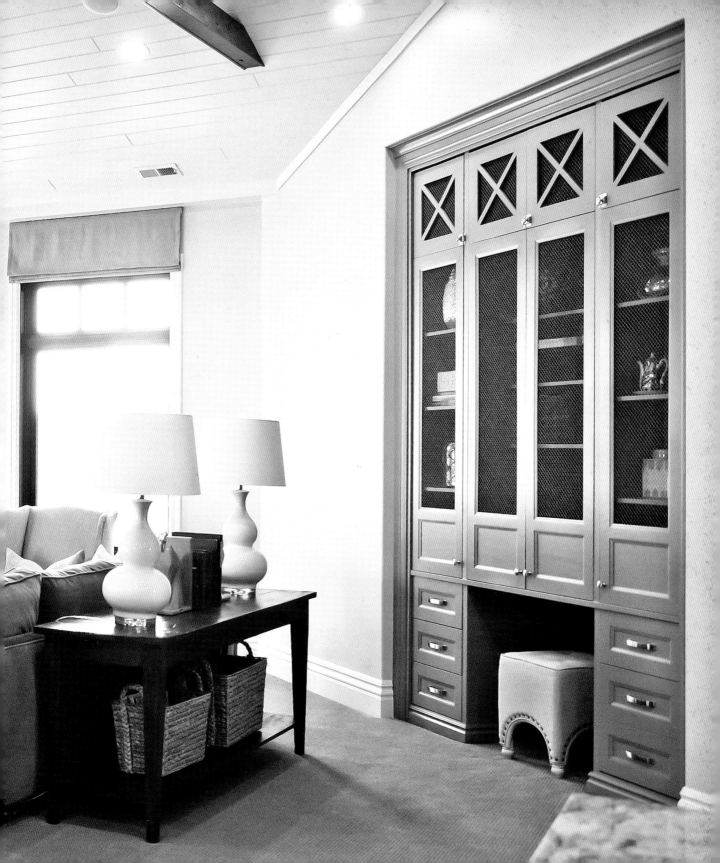

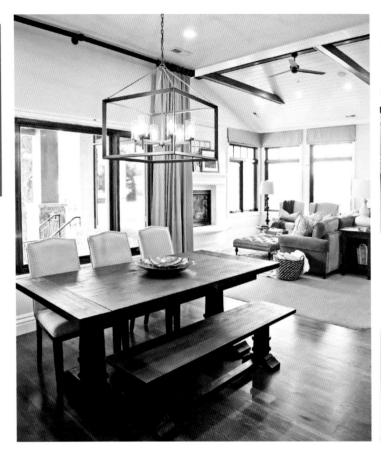

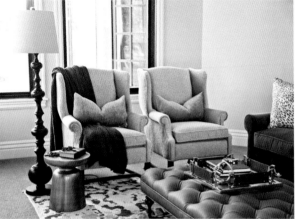

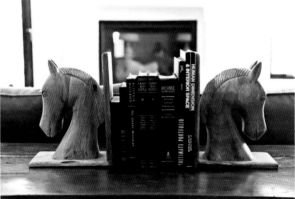

THE SIZE AND STYLE of a light fixture makes all the difference in the over-all feel of the space. Sufficient lighting is key to both setting the mood and style.

A TURNED BASE FLOOR LAMP provides reading light next to a set of wing-back chairs. A small antique brass pedestal and a supple leather otto-man provide a place to hold books or accessories.

BOOKENDS designed to mimic classic chess pieces are just one of the many unique accessories in the space.

TYING IT TOGETHER

Elements of a Sanctuary

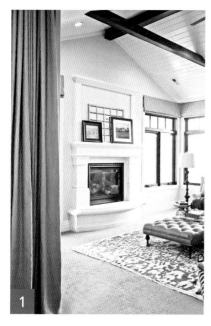 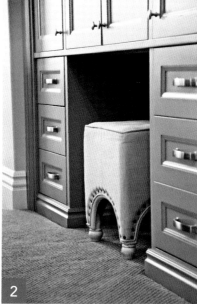 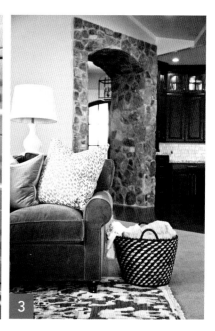

1   RICHLY STAINED WOOD BEAMS crisscross the vaulted ceiling, adding character and interest with *details and materials*.

2   BUILT-IN CABINETRY provides plenty of storage for keeping things in *order*. The cabinetry was designed to house the family computer.

3   THE GREAT ROOM opens to the adjacent dining area and kitchen, creating ample *gathering space* for family and friends.

Color and Design Principles

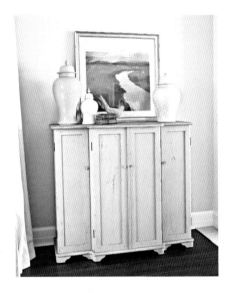

"The colors and design of a home should be
a reflection of the people who live inside."

—Amy Wax

COLOR AND DESIGN PRINCIPLES

Color is arguably the most obvious element of interior design affecting our mood and feelings. It impacts all of our human senses, including how we perceive and interpret sight, sound, taste, touch, and smell. In the design of the space, colors should be at the top of the list of careful considerations.

The six basic design principles are rhythm, balance, emphasis, harmony, proportion, and scale. Some have more of an effect on the atmosphere of a room than others, but you can get the mood you're looking for by understanding how these principles work.

Rhythm: Just as sounds or notes are arranged in a consistent pattern within a song, a repetition of design elements creates rhythm within a room. Rhythm draws the eye systematically and naturally through a space.

Balance: Our brains naturally seek balance in our environments. A well-designed space has equal visual weight of furnishings, objects, and architectural features. Balance can be symmetrical, asymmetrical, or radial.

Emphasis: Consciously drawing the eye to a dominant design feature within a space is called emphasis. Examples include a window with a beautiful view, a stately fireplace, or a grouping of art pieces. Emphasis keeps our attention focused on the things we want to highlight.

Harmony: When design features work together and complement each other to create a theme or style, a space feels harmonious. For example, you can use the same dominant colors throughout a space or include more than one furniture piece of a similar style to create harmony.

Proportion and Scale: These two design principles go hand in hand. Proportion refers to the relative size of design elements to the actual size of the space. Scale refers to the relative size of the elements to each other. For example, an oversized sofa in small living room might not feel proportionate because the size of the sofa is too big for the space. And an oversized sofa paired with a petite side chair lacks the proper relative scale to each other.

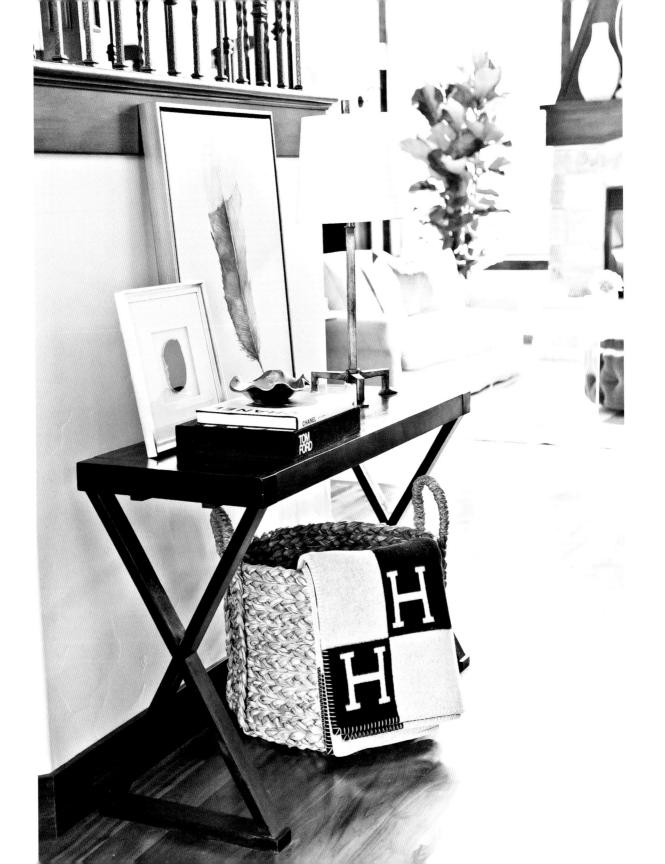

PRETTY PLEASE

Lisa Taggart wanted a sophisticated great room on the main level of her home, since the basement family room was primarily used for watching TV and lounging around. Lisa hired designer Pamela Jensen to help her tastefully replace the outdated brown tones with a fresh gray and cream palette in her ten-year-old home. Classic color and design principles were employed to make renovation a reality.

Layering various shades of gray and cream added dimension while keeping in line with Lisa's desire for a muted color palette. Pamela instinctively turned the fireplace into a focal point and relegated the television off to the side. However, this presented a design challenge. In order to keep the chairs from blocking the view of the TV, they had to be placed further back in the room, which left an immense open space between the sofa and chairs. Pam's solution was to fill the space with a long, narrow Lucite coffee table with a round ottoman tucked beneath. This combination prevented the space from feeling overwhelmed by a massive coffee table.

Because of the muted color palette, texture played an important role in the overall design. To combat a cold feeling sometimes associated with gray, Pamela maintained the home's original warm woodwork. This also helped integrate the space seamlessly into the rest of the home. A fiddle-leaf fig tree adds a touch of nature while creating balance on the opposite side of the room.

Lisa's thoroughly modern and refined space is now teeming with sophistication and elegance.

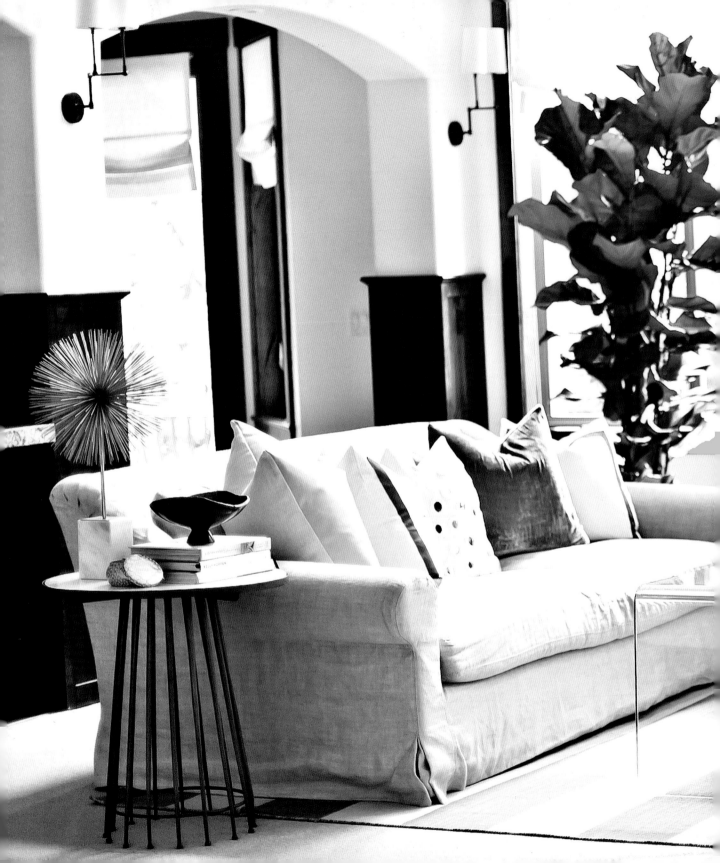

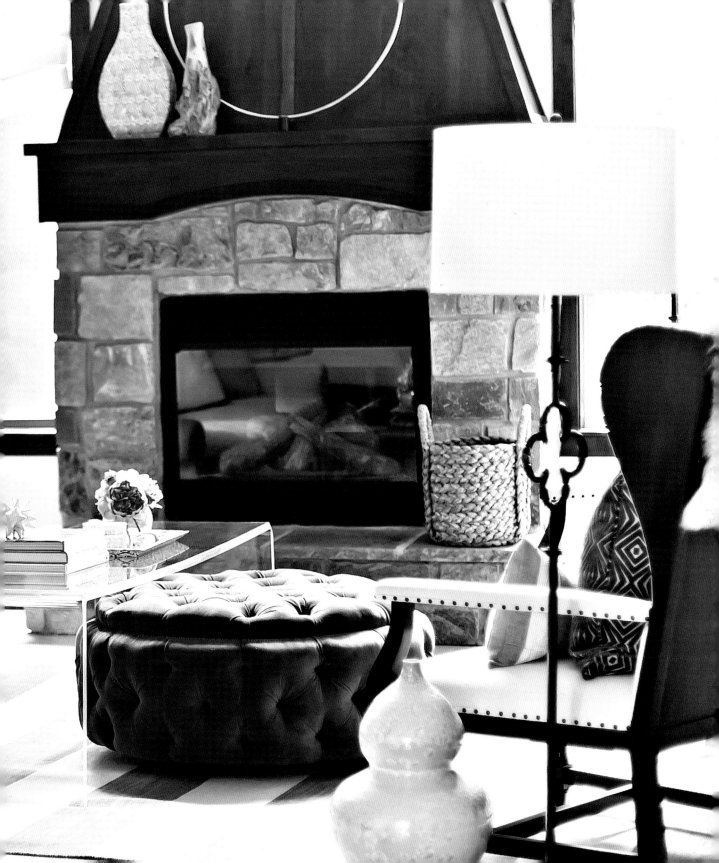

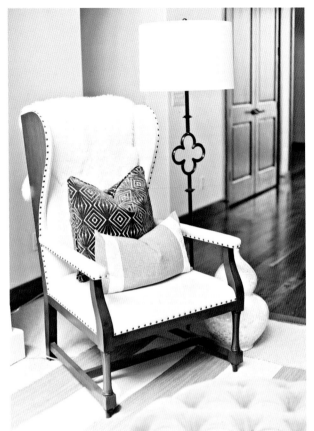

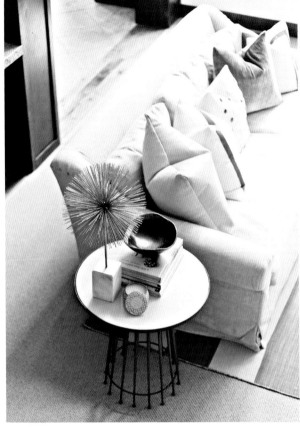

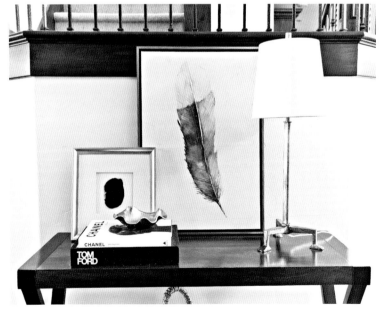

ADDING A COMFORTABLE, over-sized chair next to the television keeps the focus in the conversation area.

A SMALL ENTRY TABLE is the perfect landing spot and a welcome introduction to the adjoining room. The mixture of metals and art keeps the arrangement from feeling too formal or stuffy.

ROUND ELEMENTS keep the room from feeling overly rigid. In addition to the round end table, a natural linen sofa keeps the space casual.

TYING IT TOGETHER

Elements of a Sanctuary

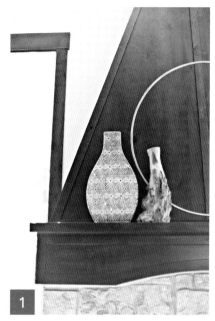
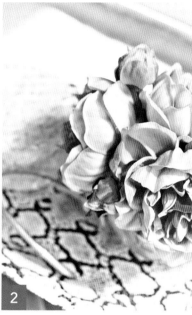
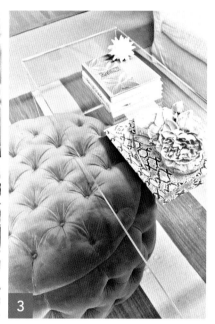

1 THE OVERSIZED brass circle represents unity, wholeness, and infinity. Placed on the center of the mantel, it creates a *symbolic* focal point.

2 THINGS THAT MATTER adorn the room, including this snakeskin tray, brass wishbone, capiz canister, and simple flower arrangement.

3 THE CLIENT'S PERSONALITY comes through in this mixture of casual elements, soft colors, and a hint of glamour.

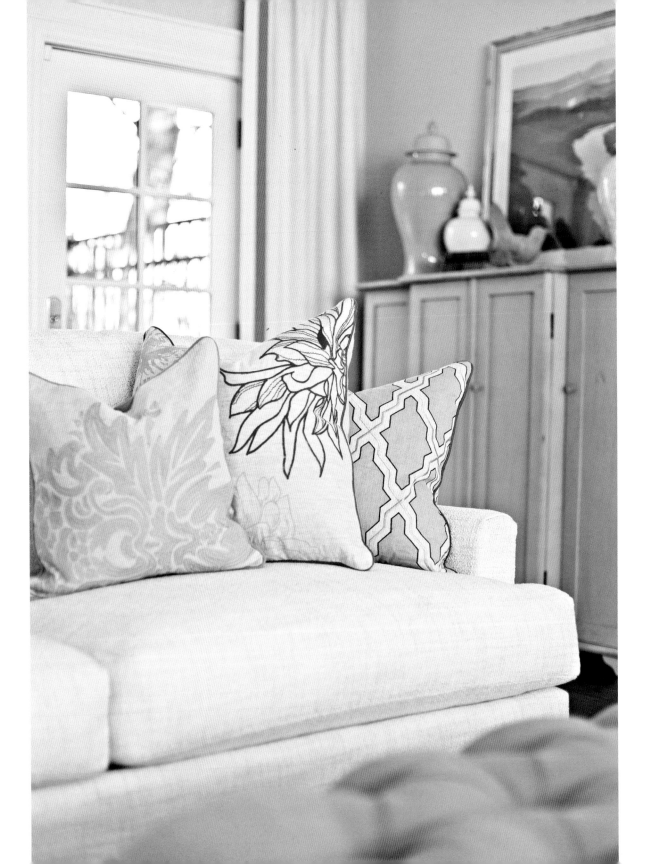

COLORFULLY CALM

Lori Radman and her family had just completed an extensive remodel and addition to their vintage home. The new space was consciously designed with a neutral color palette and uncomplicated features. When it came time to remodel the living room, however, Lori was ready for something bold.

Designer Pamela Jensen created the space to reflect Lori's style and taste, including her favorite color, coral.

A foundation of cream, light beige, and soft gray keeps the vibrant colors from overwhelming the space. A coral ottoman accentuates the seating area atop a vivacious yellow area rug. Contrasting teal accents drift throughout the room in pillows and artwork. Although the colors are vivid, they're not overly bright. This allows the room to feel rich and luxurious rather than "cutesy." Large windows immerse the space in natural light. An elegant floral oil painting on the mantel and fresh blooming branches complete the space by incorporating touches of nature.

The curious combination of coral and yellow was exactly what Lori was looking for, and it is now her favorite room in the house.

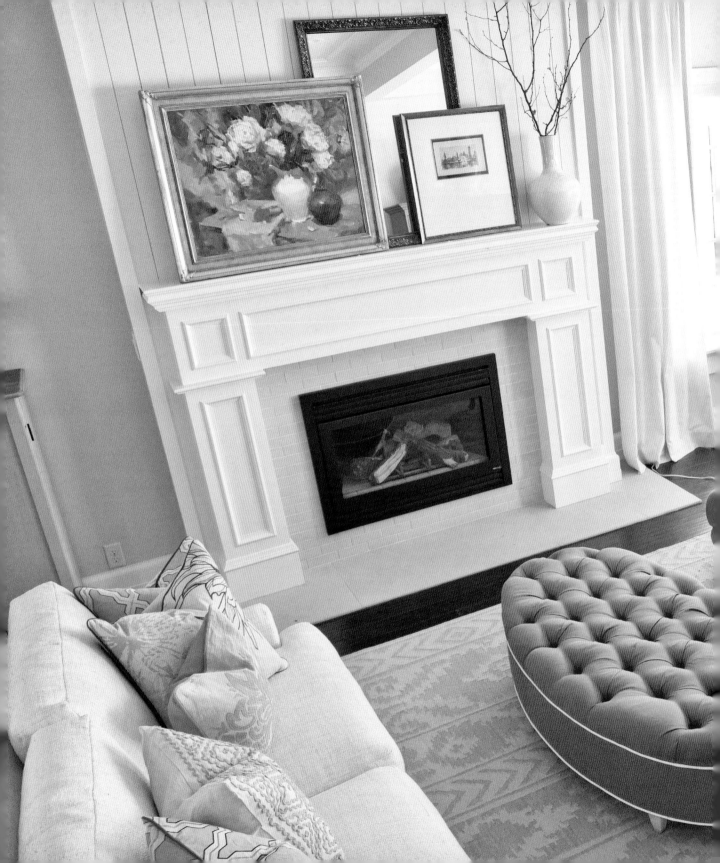

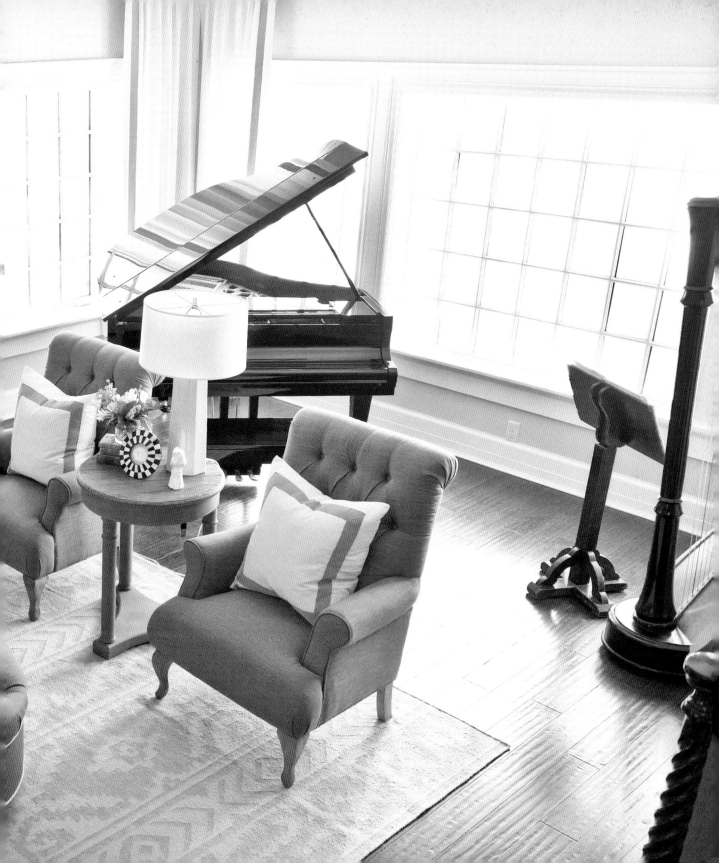

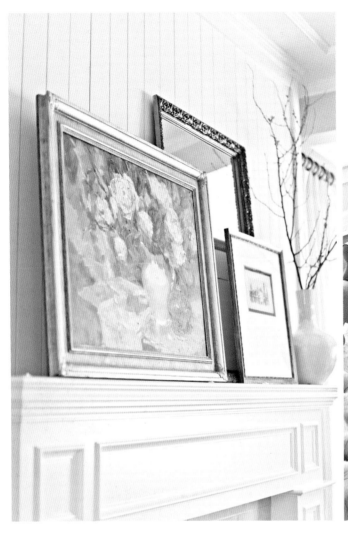

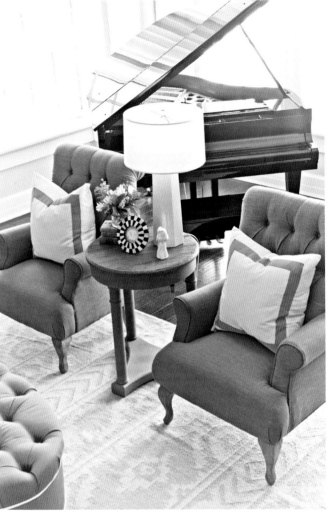

A COLLECTION OF ART and mirrors on the fireplace keep the room from feeling stuffy. The classic detailing on the white fireplace creates an elegant focal point.

A YELLOW AREA RUG grounds the space while bringing in warmth and offsetting the predominant coral accent color.

TYING IT TOGETHER

Elements of a Sanctuary

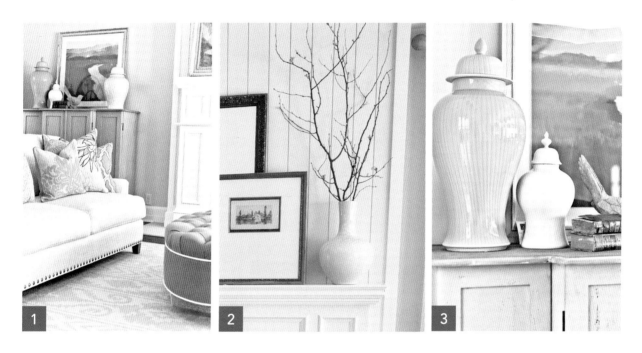

1   GROUPING THE FURNITURE and using large-scale pieces draws the room to *human scale.*

2   A SINGLE VASE filled with branches adds the element of *nature* to the space.

3   GINGER JARS in various sizes, shapes, and colors add a whimsical *detail* to the space.

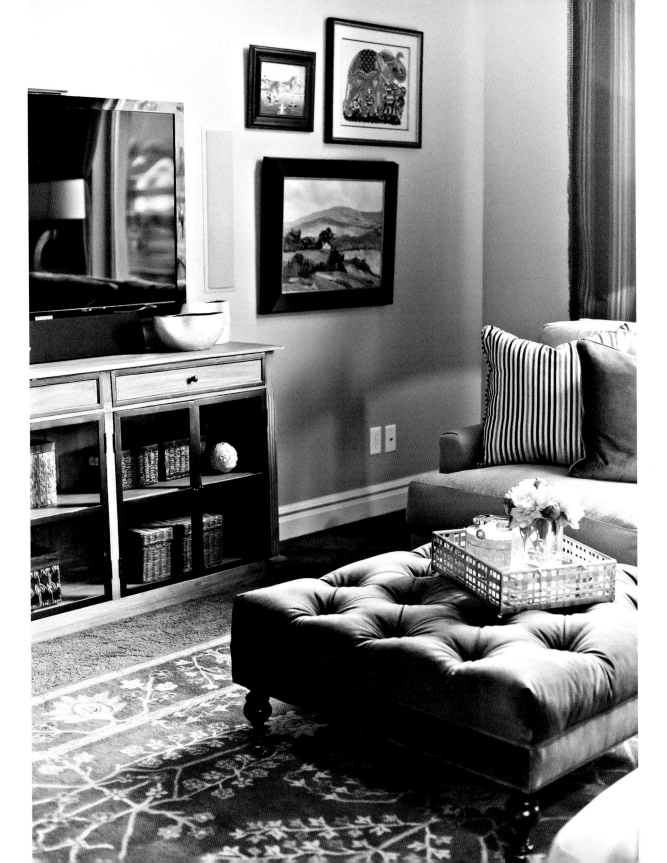

WARMING TREND

Although she couldn't put her finger on it, Theresa Call felt something was missing from her existing family room, especially her fireplace. A twenty-foot ceiling and an oversized picture window did little to create the cozy effect she was looking for.

In keeping with her clients' traditional style, the goal for designer Pamela Jensen was to pull the room in while paradoxically keeping the feel of the space open. Adding a cast stone fireplace; layering warm, rich hues; and bathing the entire space in creamy paint established the comfortable ambiance of this two-story family room.

Theresa, a world traveler, wanted to use some embroidered pillows she purchased in Turkey as her source of inspiration. From there, a rich red area rug was added in addition to other warm colors like teal and gold to tie the room together.

An oversized sectional paired with an upholstered ottoman and a dark, supple leather chair gives this room warmth and refinement. The dramatic red area rug anchors the space while also creating a sense of impact. Luxurious window treatments in a rich red hue subdue the harsh light that would typically overpower the room.

Theresa's global art collection dots the walls and finishes the space.

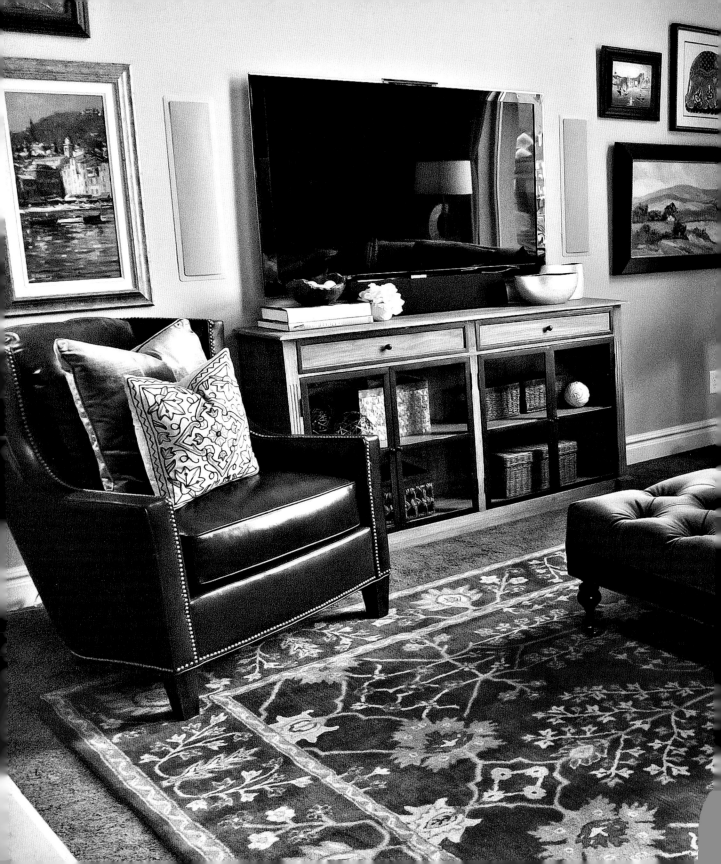

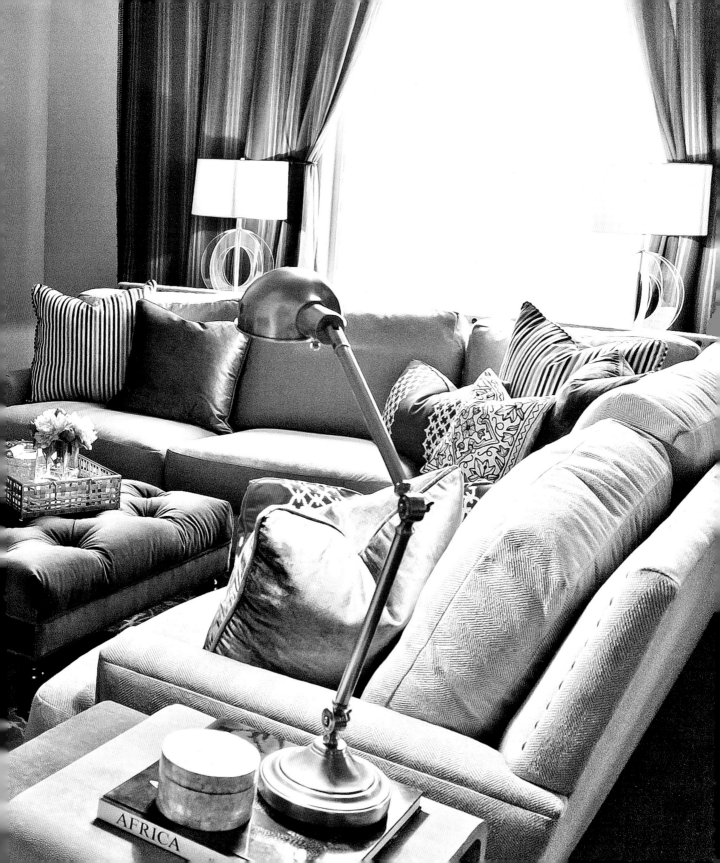

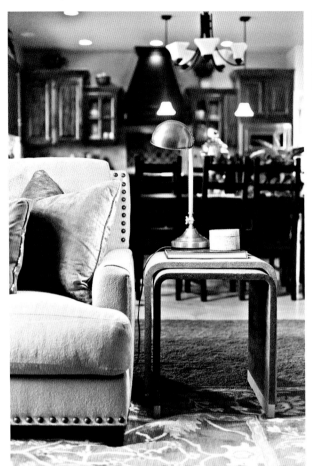

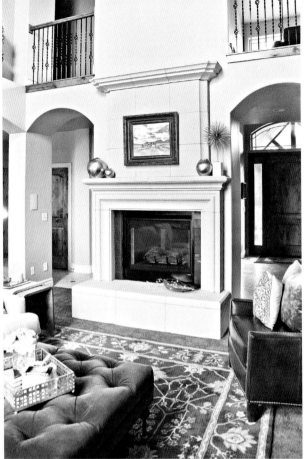

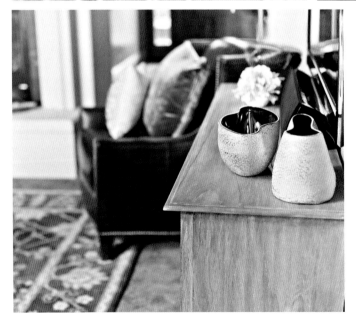

THE SIZE AND SCALE of the sofa adds visual weight. Nesting tables allow for variety in their function.

TWO-STORY ROOMS deserve a massive focal point to anchor the space and keep it from feeling lofty. In this case, designer Pamela Jensen suggested adding a cast stone fireplace.

ARTIFACTS gathered from around the world are used as decor.

TYING IT TOGETHER

Elements of a Sanctuary

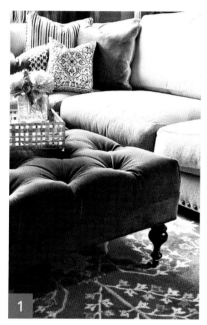
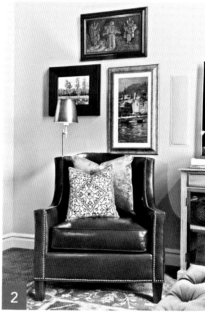
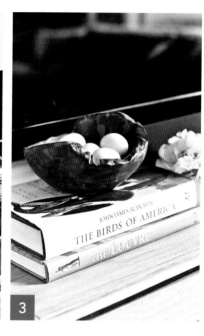

1 ADHERING TO A COMPLEMENTARY color scheme, this daring mix of red and teal shows *personality* and puts a modern spin on a traditional look. Durable textured fabrics upholster the ottoman and sofa.

2 THINGS THAT MATTER in this space include a gallery of artwork gathered from around the globe. These images are great reminders of cherished family memories and special moments in faraway places.

3 CASUAL WOOD TONES keep the room from feeling too formal for a family space. A glass cabinet display piece provides storage and adds *order* to the room.

Order

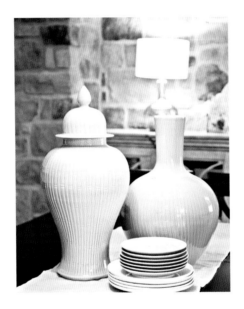

"Design is not just what it looks like and feels like. Design is how it works."

—Steve Jobs

ORDER

Environments also affect behavior and motivation. Cluttered environments attract more clutter, and a lack of productivity is the inevitable result.

Choose storage pieces whenever possible. Hidden storage is your friend! Ottomans with lift-up lids are perfect for quickly chucking in kids' toys, remote controls, and messy piles of magazines. But it doesn't stop there—instead of a side table, choose a cabinet; instead of a plain bench, pick one with under-seat storage. Sneaking in extra pockets of storage here and there throughout your home will add up to a cleaner, tidier space.

Order is a both a mental and physical function. Having order within the space creates better function with day-to-day activities. The first line of defense in tackling order is to declutter: get rid of anything that isn't beautiful or useful. This is the perfect mantra if you have difficulty deciding whether or not to let go of the "stuff" cluttering up your space. It's also a great way to decide whether or not a new purchase is a good one.

Clutter is visual distraction. Every time your eyes land on a stack of papers, a tangle of jewelry, or a pile of laundry, some small part of your mind is at work thinking about dealing with the mess. If you want a calmer experience at home, a good way to begin is by making it routine to clear all the surfaces in your house daily. When your eye can skim across clean, clear surfaces throughout your home, it also becomes easier to stay focused on the present moment. Order has a big part to play in creating the right atmosphere.

Just looking at clutter can leave you feeling stressed, overwhelmed, even depressed. And if you're a busy person and pressed for time, it can feel even more hopeless. The good news is that the process of organizing actually relieves stress and leads to great feelings of accomplishment, control, and increased self-esteem. This is why order is such a vital part of a home created to become a sanctuary.

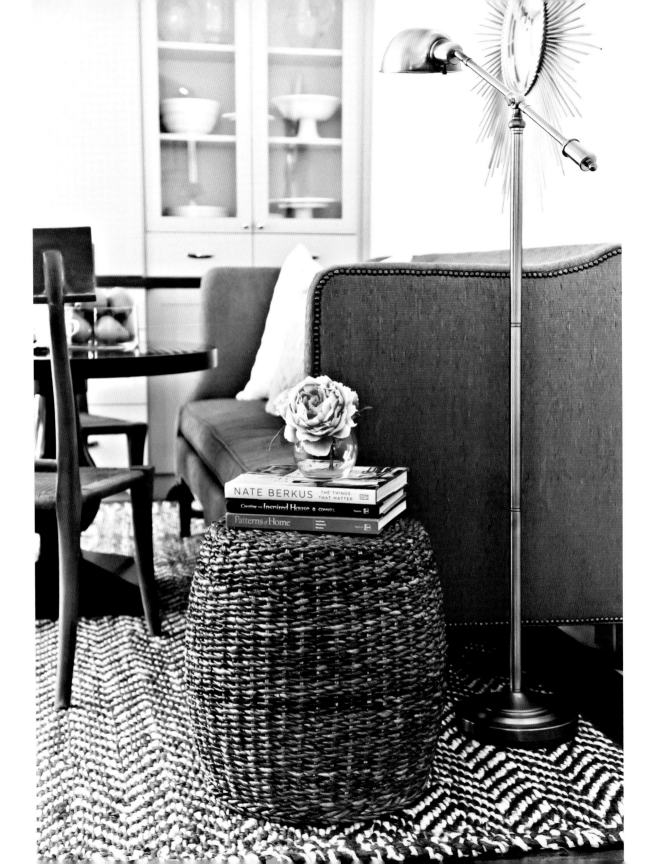

NATE BERKUS   THE THINGS
                     THAT MATTER

Creating the Inspired House B. CONNELL

Patterns of Home

ORDER IN THE HOUSE

The sunlit room adjacent to Kristy Feller's great room and kitchen was a quaint pocket of unused space begging to be transformed into a multipurpose study room. Wall-to-wall french doors and a bank of windows steep the room in natural light. The prime location of the room, relative to the heart of the home, makes it a perfect in-between space.

Designer Deboni Sacre's first impression was to design a multifunctional built-in cabinet to provide storage for an assortment of items, including everything from servingware to a home computer. The cabinet was designed with glass fronts and recessed lighting to showcase elegant items and with oversized doors to hide the computer and its components.

A comfortable settee serves for different activities—providing seating for the small tea table during an informal meal or for use as part of a conversation area. An easy-to-care-for fabric covers the settee and stands up well in a household with four growing boys. A decorative mirror above the settee reflects the natural light and view of nature from the opposite wall.

Creamy white and soft gray are the foundation of this space while warm, metallic accents add a bit of contrast. A perfectly scaled pendant light above the table provides a mix of ambient and task lighting.

To complete the look, a hint of pink was added for this busy mom who lives in a house ruled by boys.

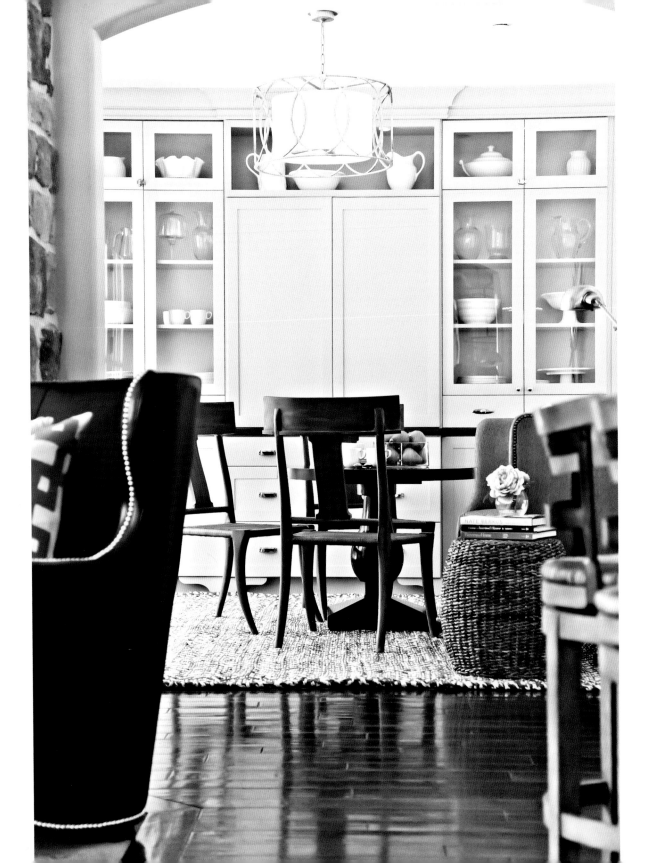

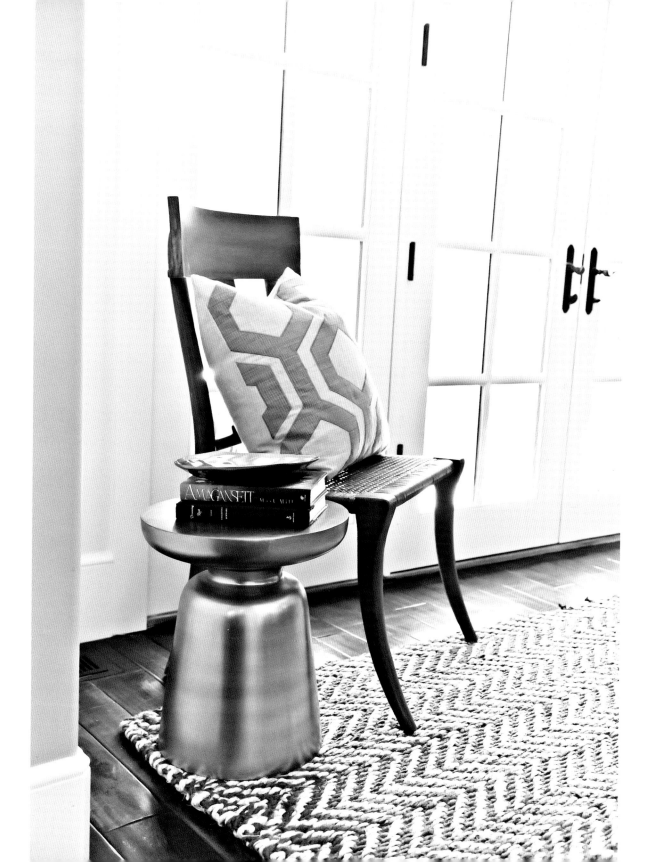

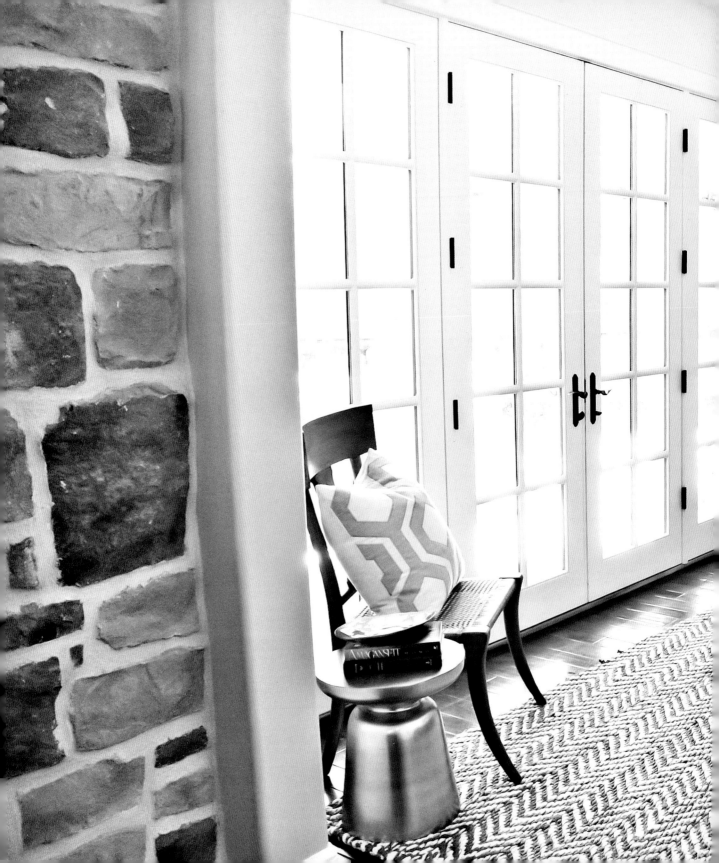

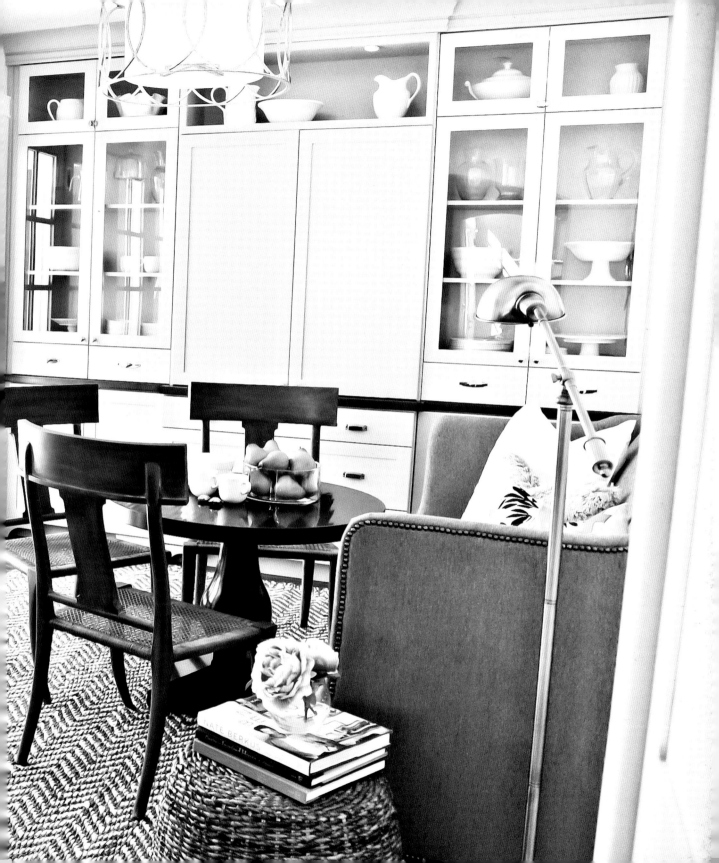

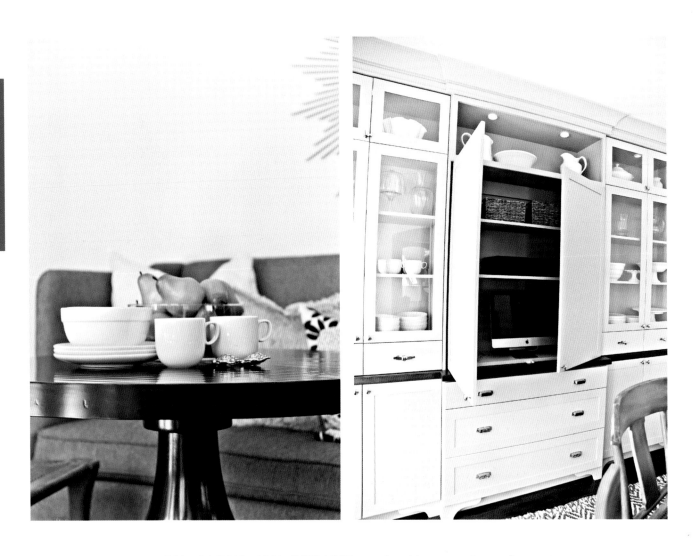

FOR CASUAL AND INTIMATE meals, this room is perfect. The small table also doubles as a second homework spot.

DEBONI DESIGNED the cabinet to hide away the components when not in use.

TYING IT TOGETHER

Elements of a Sanctuary

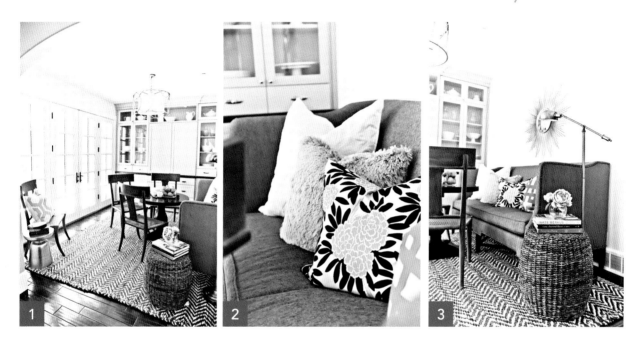

1 WARMTH AND NATURAL LIGHT fill the room from the wall of windows and doors opposite the sofa creating a connection to *nature* in this room. The sisal rug and jute table also add elements of nature.

2 SOFT TONES of grey and putty are the perfect background for a hint of *color*. The subtlety of color keeps the room feeling classic and restful.

3 GLASS DOORS, shining metals, and sparkling mirrors create a feeling of *inspiration* in an environment. The room is a perfect place to feel lifted by thought, music, or literature.

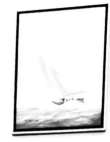
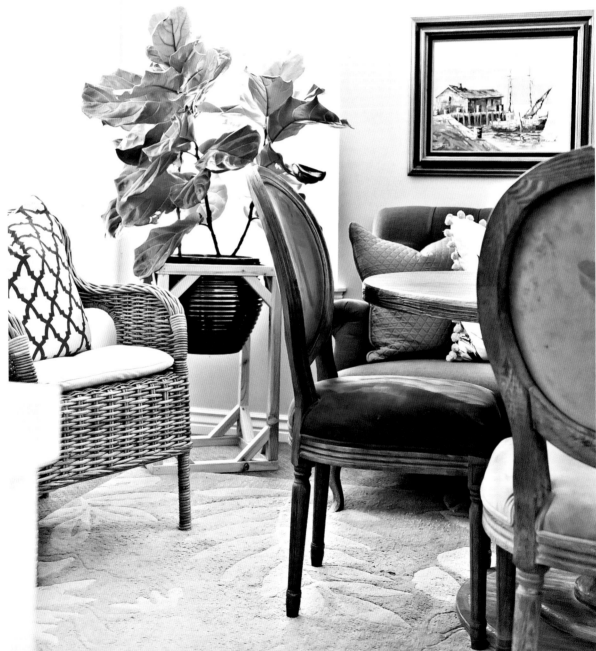

ROOM WITH A HUE

Christy Petrie was looking for a multifunctional space that could be integrated into her new home. Since she homeschools her four children, she wanted to convert an underused, secluded room into a functional and fun space for school and music. Christy's first priority was to provide ample desk space with seating for four, and built-in bookshelves with storage for musical instruments.

Because of the small space, designer Pamela Jensen had a real challenge on her hands. She needed to meet all of the family's needs and make the room still feel inviting. Since the children would spend lots of time in the room, it was important to make it feel pleasant.

The first task was designing built-ins with columns that added function and some separation from the entry. The built-ins create order for books and school supplies. Next on Pam's design list was to create a furniture plan to accommodate the functional needs of the room. The key to this successful design is a petite settee that provides comfortable seating at the round table used as a school desk. Three additional chairs surround the school table to accommodate all the children. A couple of extra chairs are tucked in the corner for extra seating opposite the piano.

Bright colors and decorative accents make this cozy little space an ideal and functional workspace.

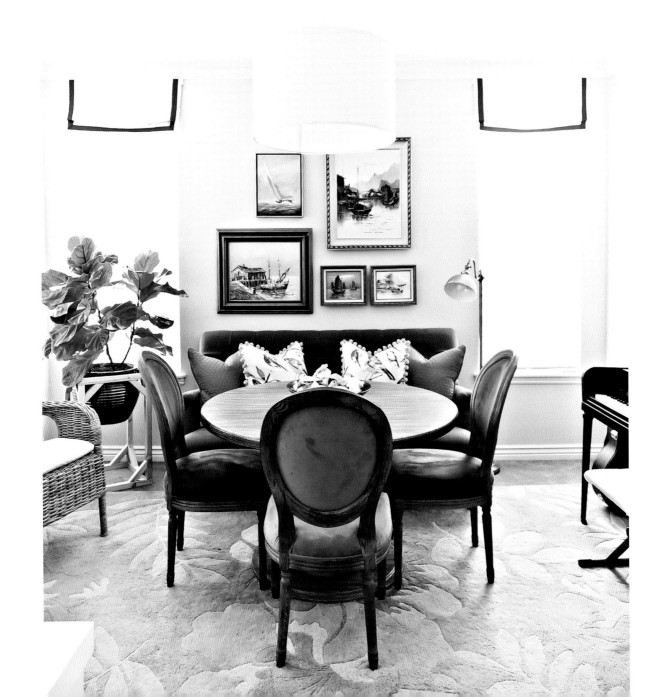

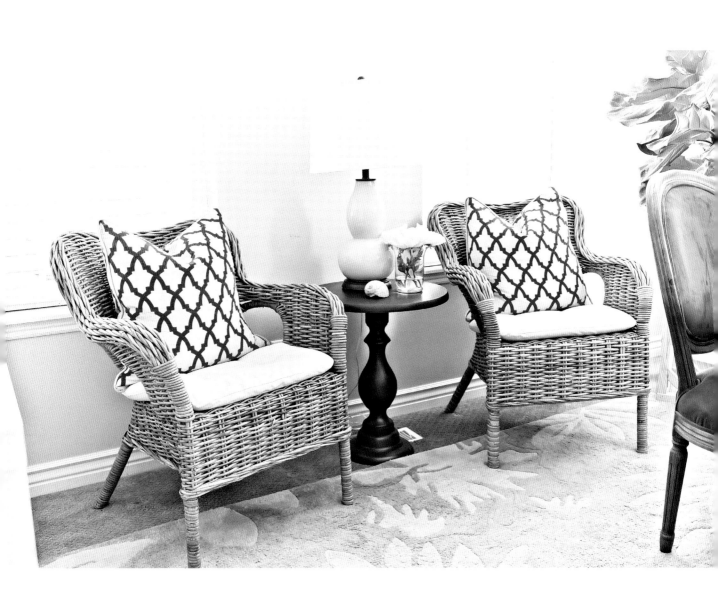

A COMFORTABLE SETTEE with soft and bright pillows creates the perfect spot in this unique room for doing homework.

SEMI-OPEN BUILT-IN BOOKSHELVES serve as a subtle room divider and separate the work zone from the rest of the house.

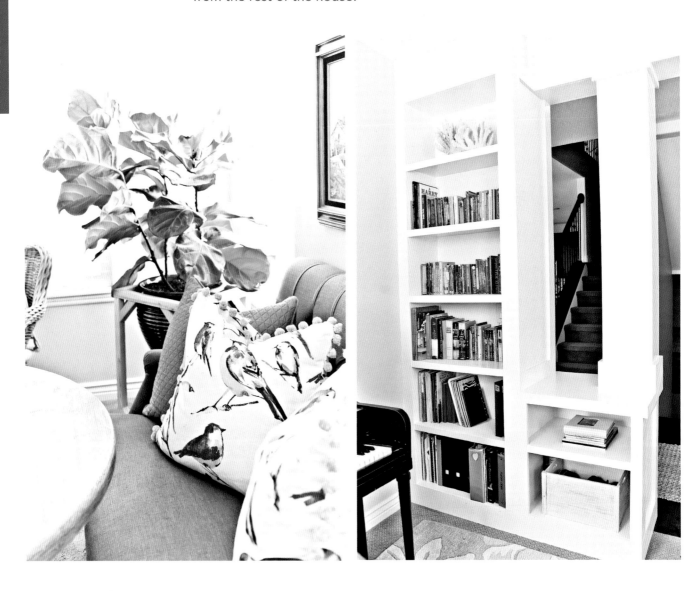

TYING IT TOGETHER

Elements of a Sanctuary

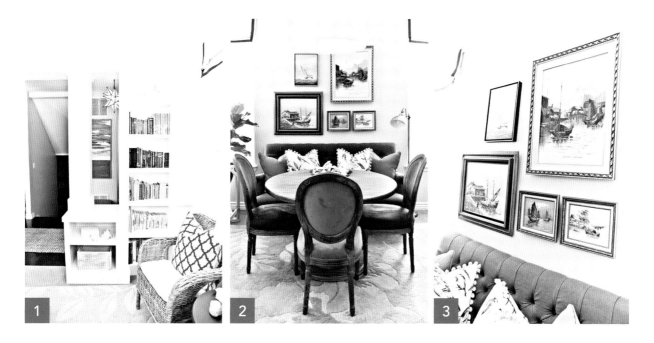

1   BOOKSHELVES AND COLUMNS symmetrically mirror the room entry and bring the design principle of balance. The unique design adds *detail* to both the homework room and entry.

2   VIBRANT TEAL CHAIRS highlight the worktable and various elements throughout the room. Studies have shown that bright *colors* enhance productivity.

3   THINGS THAT MATTER include coastal artwork, seashells, and coral displayed throughout the room—remnants of happy times when the family lived on the East Coast.

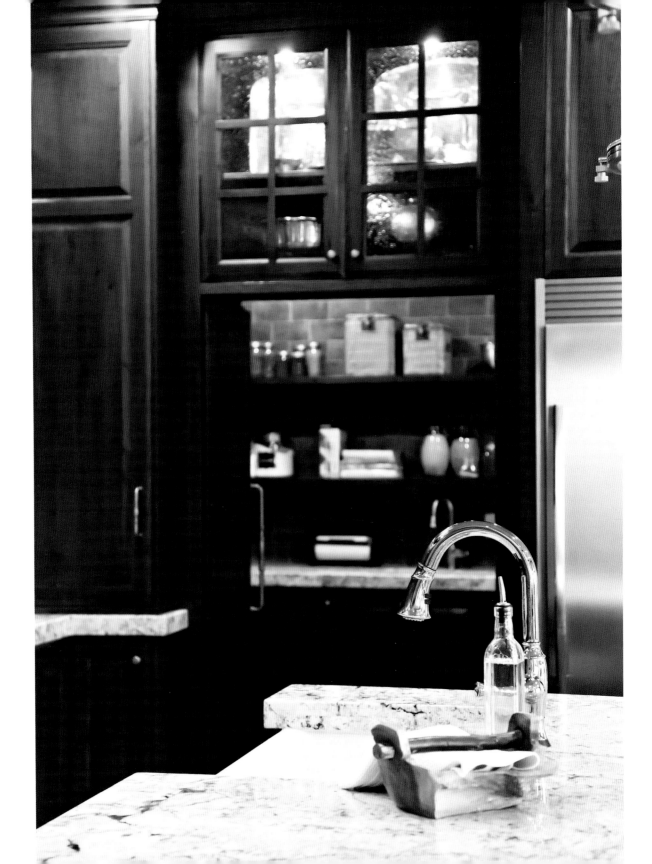

PRETTY AND PRACTICAL

Organization and aesthetics in a kitchen are an obvious must, and designer Pamela Jensen, teaming with homeowner Rachelle Olsen, accomplished just that for this busy family of six. The successful design of this hard-working kitchen has a place for everyone and everything.

Attention to detail is the key component that makes this kitchen work. Dishes, baking pans, servingware and utensils each have designated storage space, which makes it easy for quick access while preparing and serving meals. Glass upper cabinets reveal a cherished silver and pewter collection, and a recessed paper towel holder in the island maximizes countertop space.

However, the key ingredient of this smart and stylish kitchen is the walk-in pantry. Double doors lead into the pantry, which houses small, unsightly appliances like the microwave and toaster. A full-size freezer also finds its home here, separate from the refrigerator in the kitchen area. The pantry keeps these kitchen essentials tucked away yet conveniently located.

The layout and look of the space incorporates everything Rachelle was looking for. The result is a perfect combination of fresh and functional living.

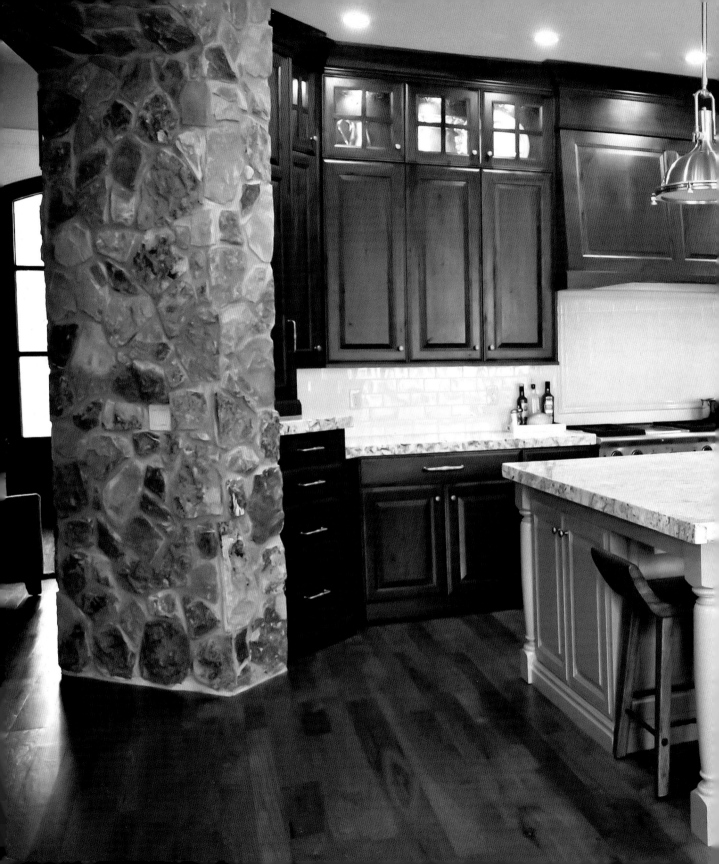

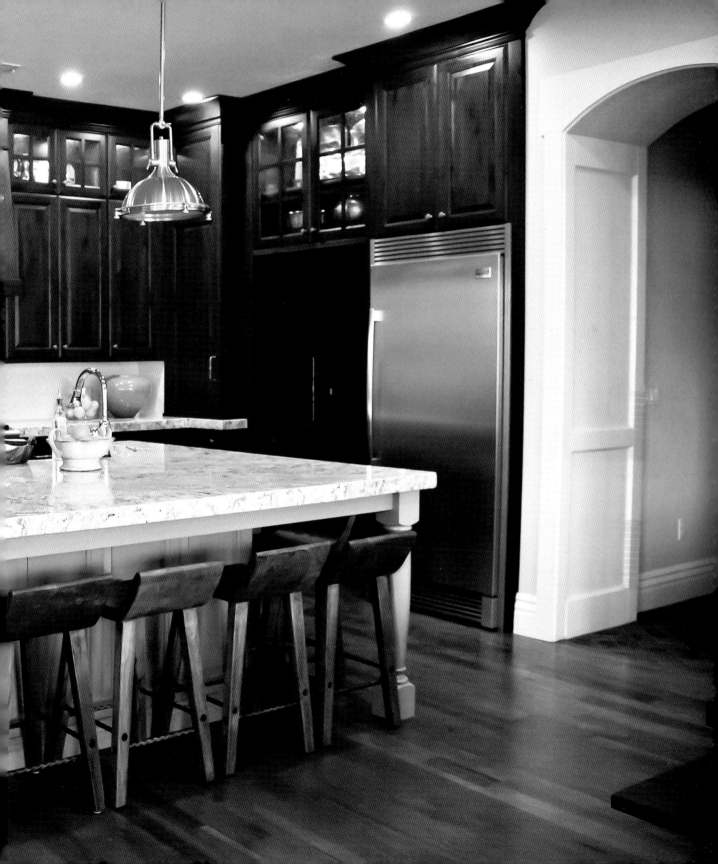

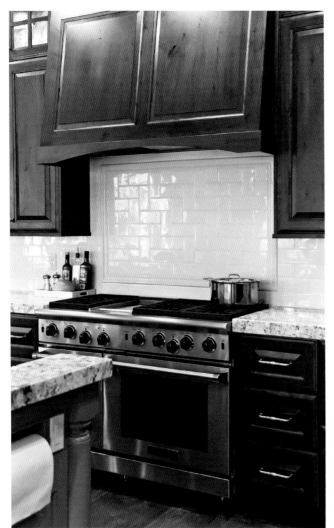

EVERY INCH OF THE CUSTOM CABINETRY offers storage, including the island's recessed paper towel holder.

CLEVER STORAGE COMPARTMENTS were added throughout the kitchen. A pullout drawer conveniently stores kitchen utensils.

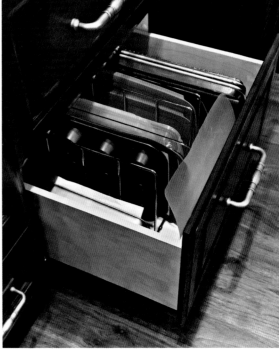

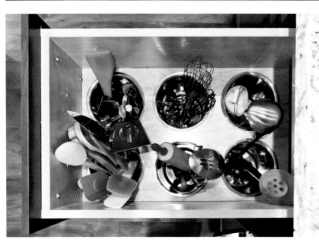

TYING IT TOGETHER

Elements of a Sanctuary

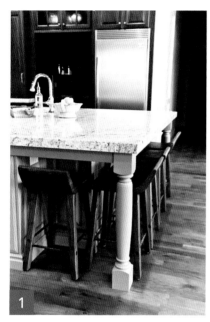
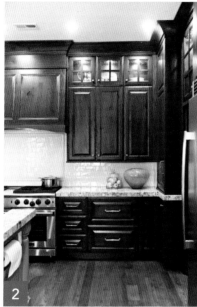
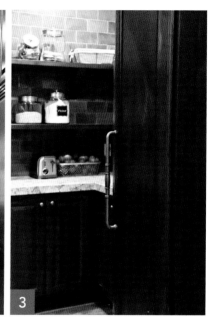

1   IN THIS GATHERING SPACE, an oversized island provide ample seating for family and friends.

2   GLOSSY SUBWAY TILES, glass-front cabinets and a light granite counter-top enhance the ambient *light* in this space.

3   THE WALK-IN PANTRY was designed as a cabinet-framed room transition. An exposed brick wall highlights the open shelving and is a unique use of *details and materials.*

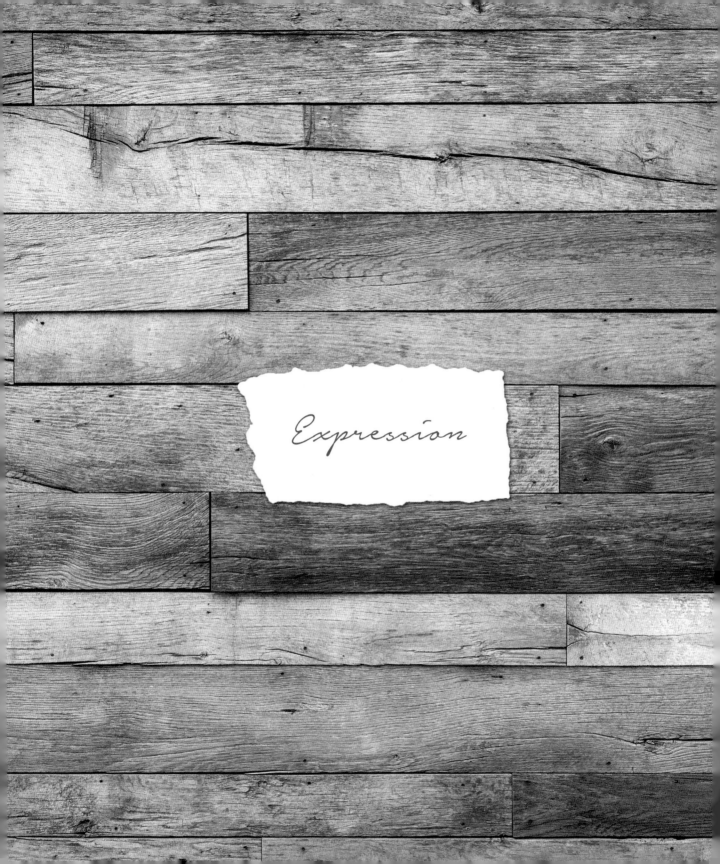

Expression

EXPRESSION

Your home is a reflection of who you are. It is infused with your essence, your character, and your spirit. When we express ourselves in our homes, we project our sense of self to the world around us. Our heritage, our interests, our likes and dislikes are all reflected in the space we inhabit, whether we do it intentionally or not. Self-expression is one of the most basic human needs. What better place to showcase it than in our homes?

Color, style, and decor all reflect our personality. Bright colors tend to energize and inspire, while muted colors soothe and comfort. When the foundation of a room, including the floors, walls, and ceilings, are designed with a neutral palette, introduce bright or bold color through furniture and accessories, which can easily be changed out over time.

Our home is the best place to use as a creative outlet. It's a safe place to try out different ideas in various rooms while we show off different parts of our personality.

Interior Reflection

ASK YOURSELF THE FOLLOWING QUESTIONS WHEN CONTEMPLATING
THE **EMOTIONAL ATMOSPHERE** OF YOUR HOME:

1. Does the space reflect the truth of who I am or who I want to be?
2. What do I most connect with? Why? How can it be incorporated into the design?
3. What would give my space more meaning?
4. How do the architectural details influence the overall design?
5. Are the materials used in the space reflective of the feeling I'd like to create?

Personality

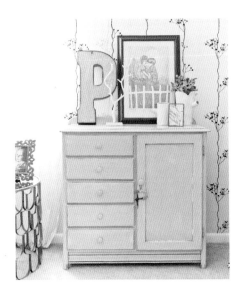

"Style is a way to say who you are
without having to speak."

—Rachel Zoe

PERSONALITY

Color, style, and decor, including furniture and accessories, all reflect our personality within a space. Bright colors tend to energize and inspire, while muted colors soothe and comfort. When the foundation of a room, including the floors, walls and ceilings, are designed with a neutral palette, introduce bright or bold color through accents, which can easily be changed out over time.

Establishing a particular style is easier when it's based on a set of parameters. These parameters are usually based on an era in time like Victorian or American Colonial; a style of art or furniture such as Art Deco or Industrial; or a lifestyle such as Sophisticated or Urban. Whichever style you choose to reflect in your surroundings says a lot about your personality.

The types of furniture and accessories we choose also reflect our personality. For example, clean lines and muted colors convey a sense of sophistication, while a playful atmosphere is filled with eclectic items and a bolder color palette.

When creating a sanctuary, the important thing is to let your personality shine through your surroundings.

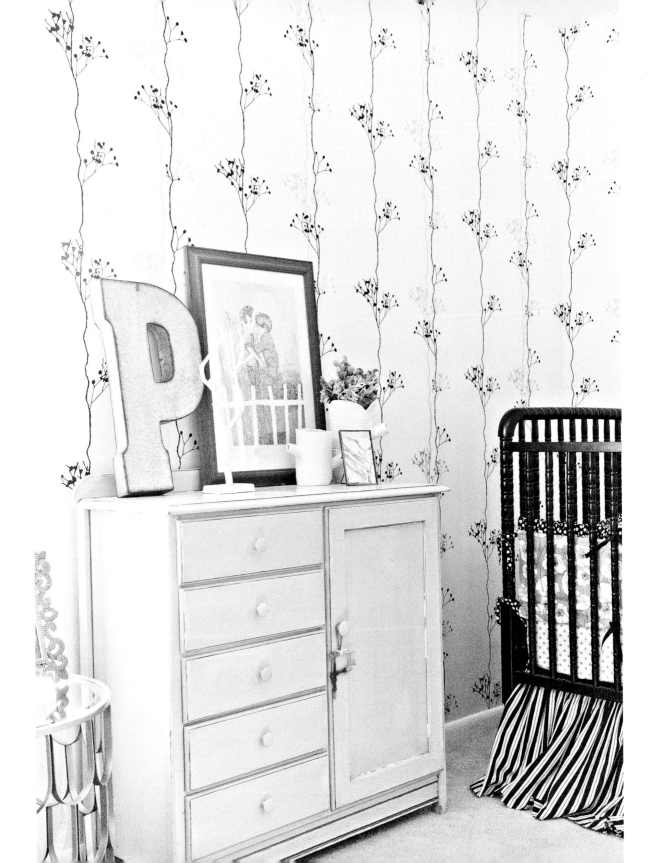

P IS FOR PRECIOUS

P is also for Penny, the adorable daughter of Liv Showroom designer Sam Zenger. Fortunately for Penny, her talented mother designed this eclectic wonderland to accommodate future growth or the addition of a sibling.

Sam's goal was to design a functional nursery . . . emphasis on the *fun*. The liberal mix of colors combined with black and white accents makes the color palette versatile enough for either a girl or a boy. The home was built in 1946, so Sam wanted to honor the decor of the era while bringing it into modern times.

A Coty Airspun loose-face-powder box Sam remembered from her childhood was the inspiration behind the art-deco-themed space. Sam used a creamy orange poppy fabric for the bumper pads, and from there she added retro touches throughout.

An original Milo Baughman recliner is the perfect mid-century addition, while being functional for nighttime feedings and bedtime routines. The scalloped metallic side table adds a touch of funky detail without taking up too much space next to the large solid dresser. An adjustable arm lamp provides directional lighting and is a stylish alternative to a traditional table lamp. Sheer window panels loosely drape the windows and soften the space while disguising blackout roller shades beneath.

The antiquated mix of materials, fabrics, and colors exclaims personality, charm, and character.

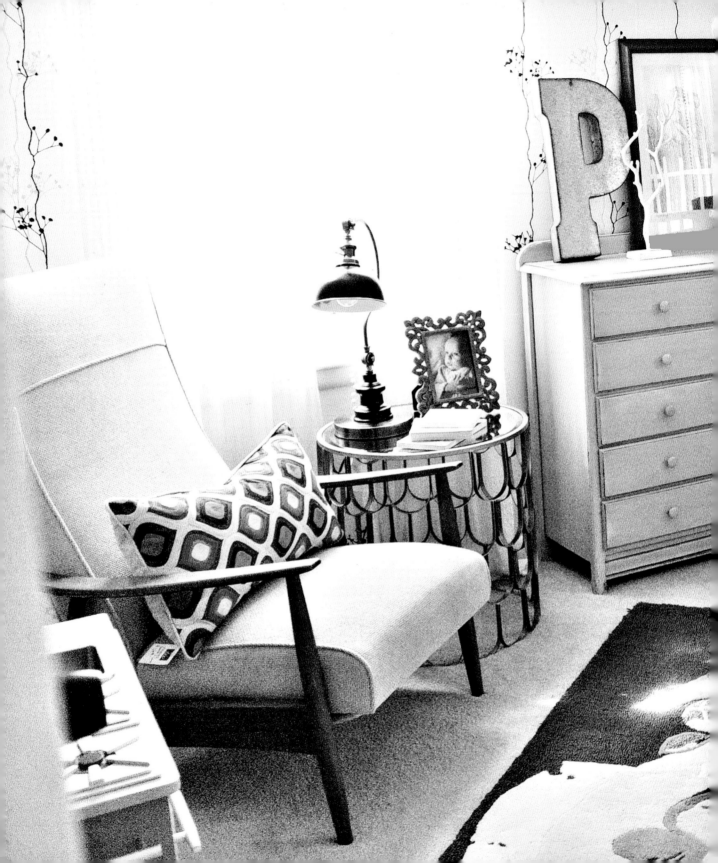

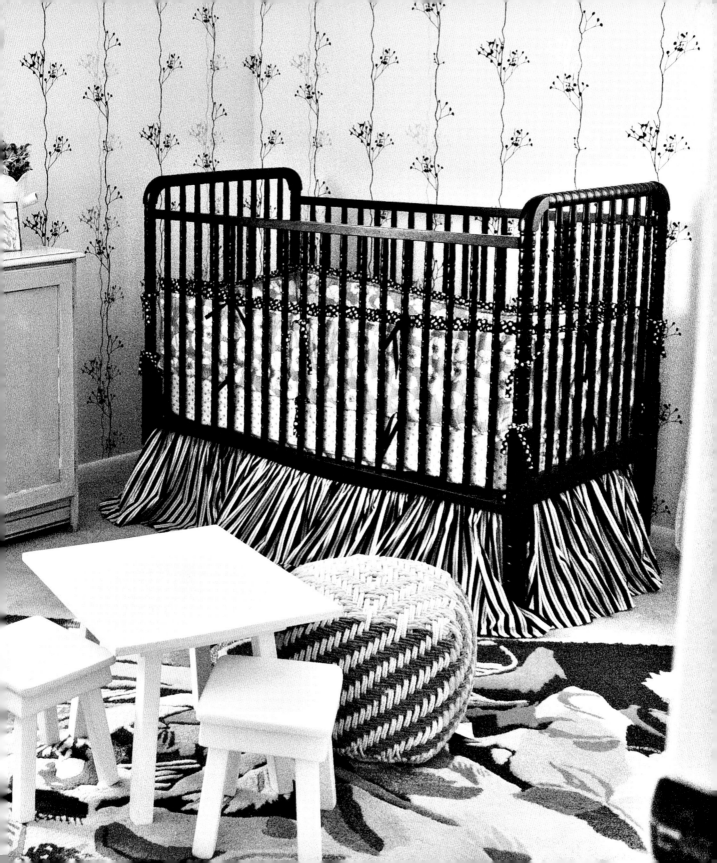

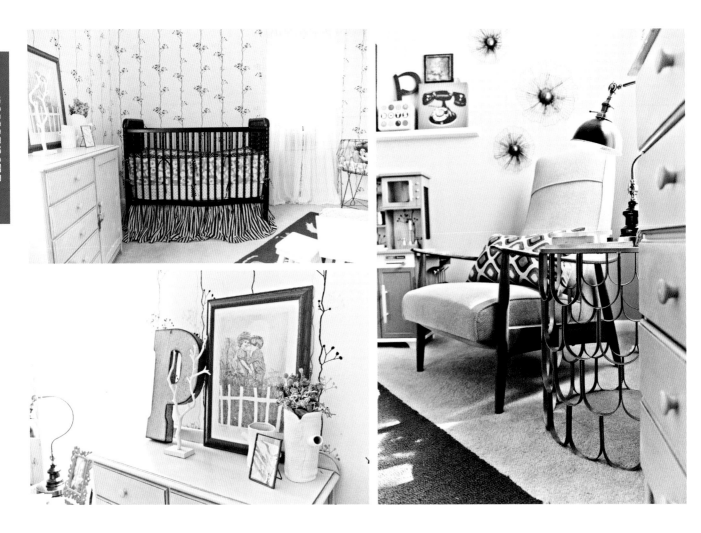

A SIMPLISTIC FLORAL PATTERN climbs up the walls, and a black and white bed skirt puddles beneath the crib, mimicking the flow of the pattern in the wallpaper.

RETRO DETAILS include a Milo Baughman recliner, Sputnik-inspired wall art, and a restored vintage play kitchen.

TYING IT TOGETHER

Elements of a Sanctuary

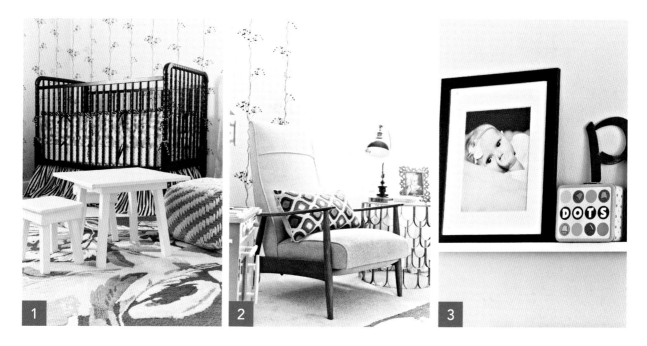

1 A FUN RUG with an oversized graphic pattern adds interest while bringing in *color* and design principles.

2 ADDING A CHAIR to a quiet corner in any room is the perfect spot for *private space.*

3 THINGS THAT MATTER are artfully displayed on simple wall shelf. Beloved treasures, pictures, and art can easily be updated as the room evolves over time.

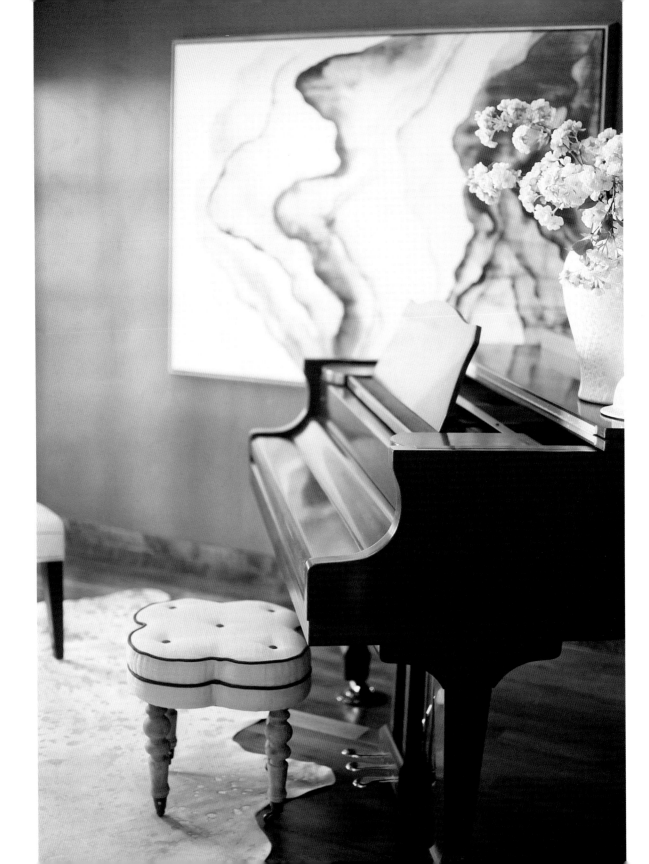

MUSIC TO MY EARS, BEAUTY TO MY EYES

The music room is the first room guests see when they enter Lisa Taggart's house; therefore, she wanted this space to make a bold statement. Lisa and designer Pamela Jensen worked together to create a room full of personality with a touch of glamour.

Lisa and Pamela chose a saturated color for the walls to emphasize the dramatic artwork and create an emotional feeling in the space. The choice of colors and materials differentiate it from the neutral palette in the rest of the house.

The organic shape of a metallic cowhide rug mimics the movement in the artwork. Formal seating stands opposite of a classic grand piano.

The juxtaposition of dark and light and formal and informal are a perfect reflection of Lisa's personality and style.

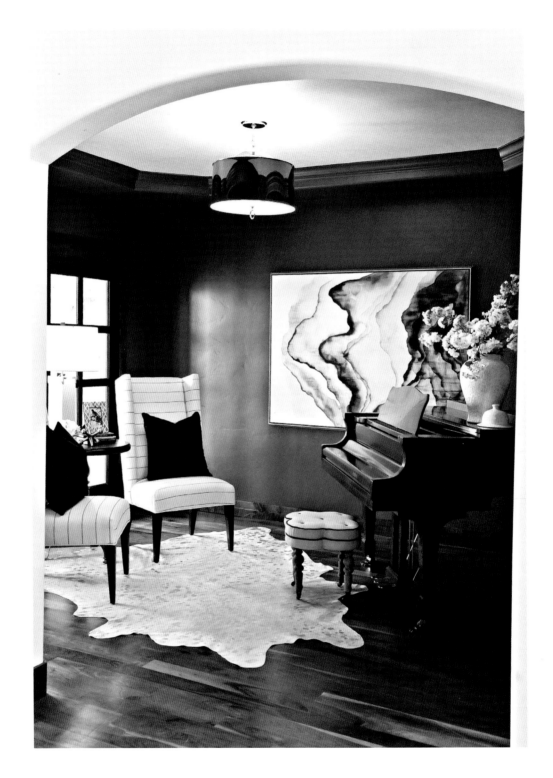

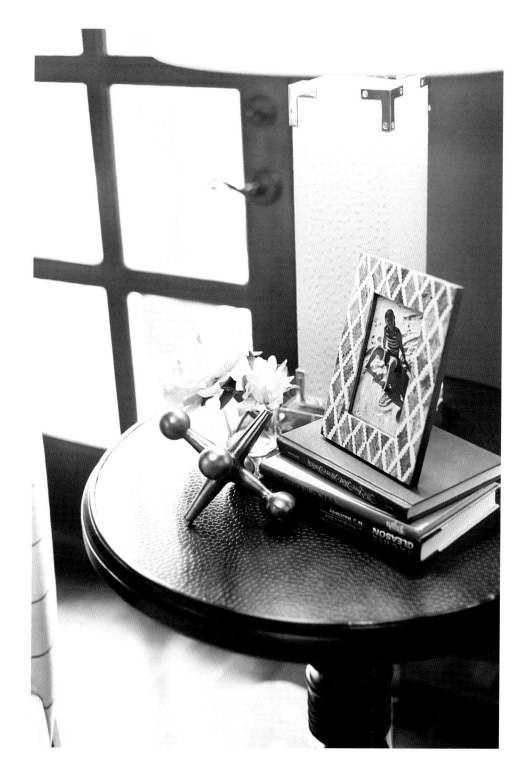

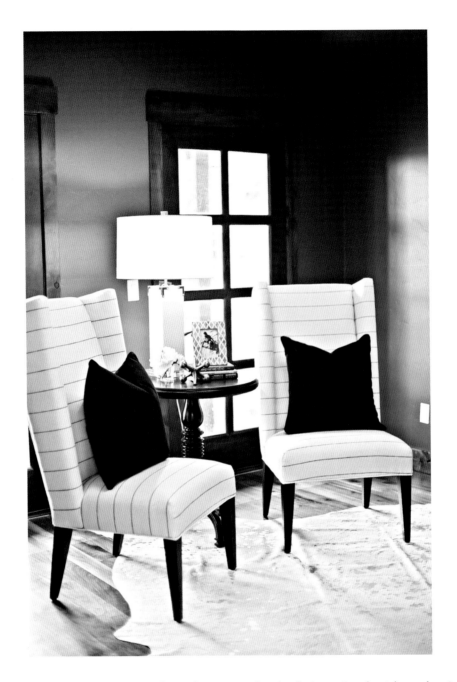

STRIKING ARTWORK and modern wing-back chairs mixed with a classic grand piano create high contrast, showcasing Lisa's personality.

TYING IT TOGETHER

Elements of a Sanctuary

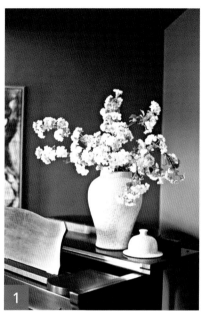 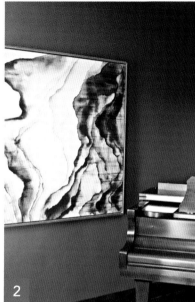 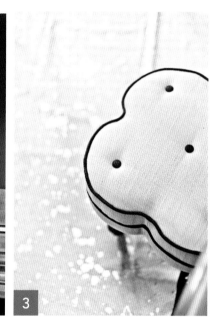

1   A SMALL FLORAL arrangement adds a touch of *nature* and keeps the room from feeling too stuffy.

2   INSPIRATIONAL, EYE-POPPING artwork creates emphasis and a focal point, an important *design principle*.

3   A TRADITIONAL piano stool is traded out for this whimsical stool with contrasting piping. A metallic cowhide rug adds an elegant shimmer to this *in-between space*.

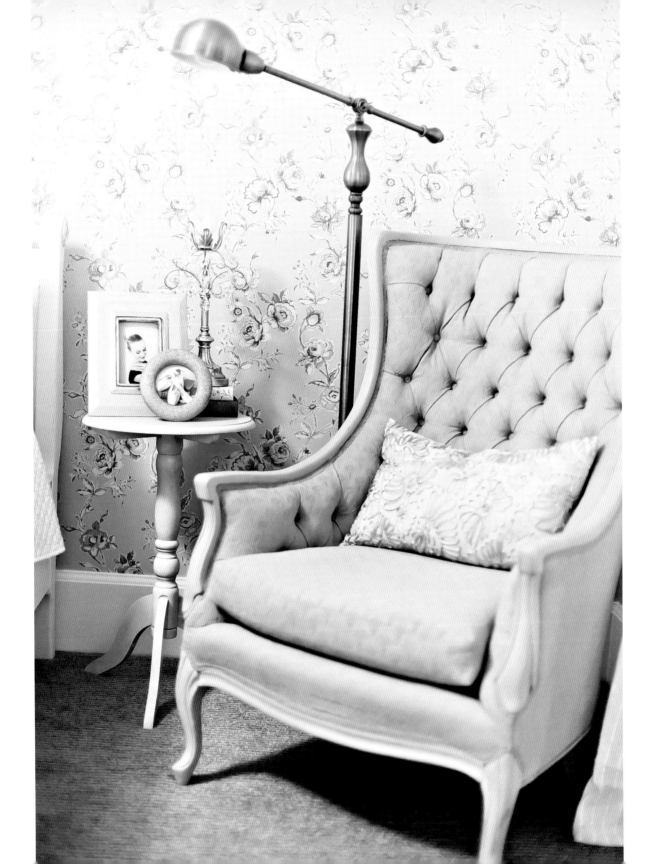

PRETTY IN PINK

When thirteen-year-old Kayla Krstic's family built a new home recently, her parents promised she could decorate her bedroom however she wanted. Fortunately, with a little direction from designer Tonya Olsen and a guiding hand from mom Christine, Kayla created a dreamy sanctuary full of soft pastels, elegant fabrics and sentimental keepsakes fitting for a teenage girl.

Despite the popularity of bold colors and modern furnishings so often seen in teenage bedrooms these days, Kayla preferred the look of a vintage retreat. Her love of ballet can be seen throughout the room in framed pictures and dance-related decor.

Kayla chose a classic floral wallpaper to highlight the wall behind her antique bed. She updated a tufted accent chair that had been passed down in the family with a fresh coat of paint to both the fabric and the frame. Kayla's bedding is simple yet comfortable with an assortment of throw pillows that add texture, color, and variety. To balance the wallpaper on the opposite wall, Kayla hung a gallery of carved mirrors, vintage plates, and antique doorknobs. A traditional vanity doubles as a small desk for Kayla to sit at and do homework.

Kayla's personality is perfectly reflected in this dreamy sanctuary.

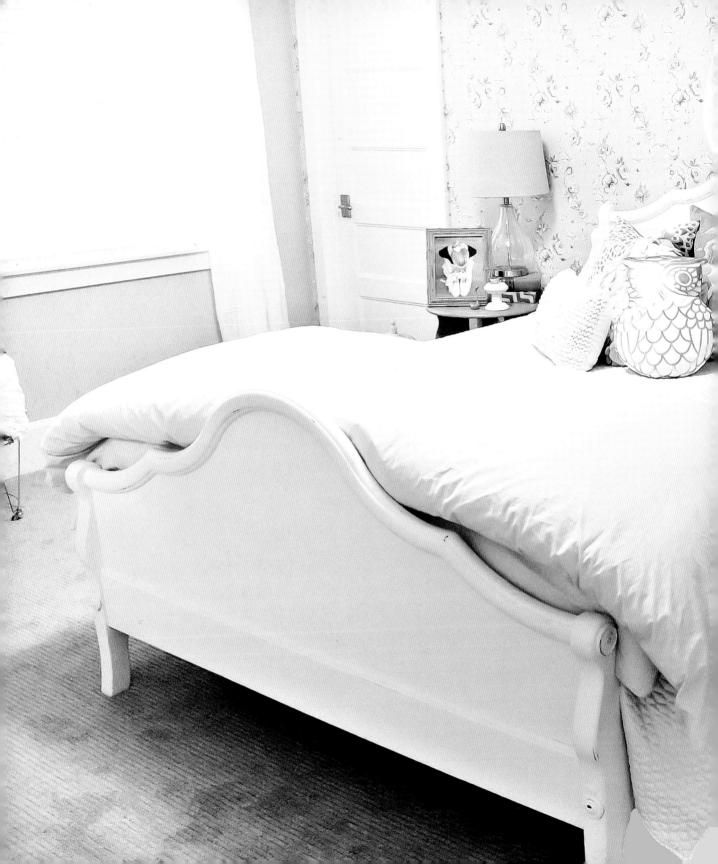

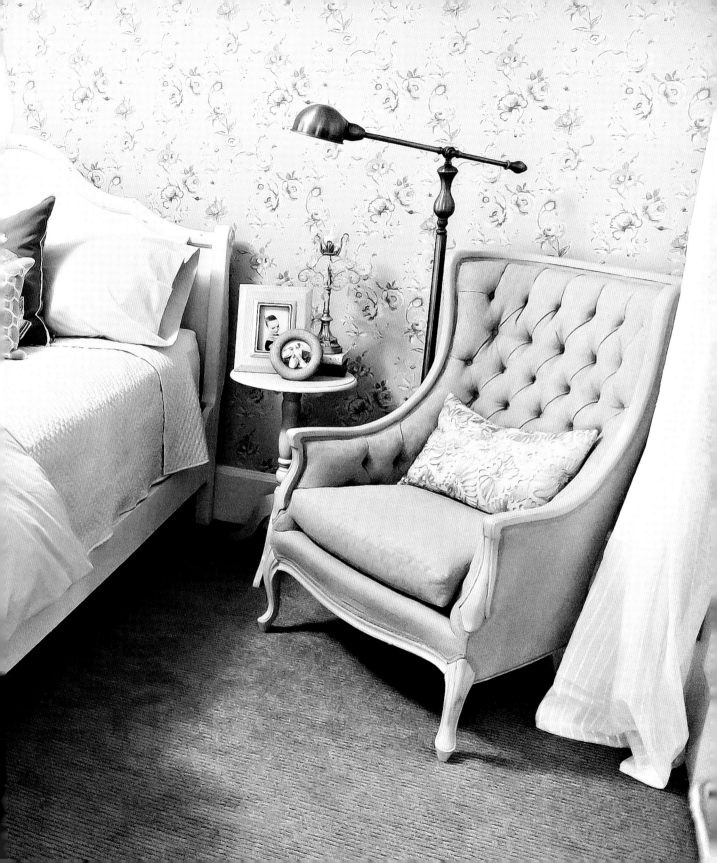

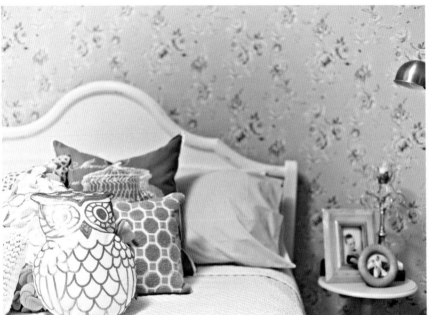

A MIXTURE OF THROW pillows in a variety of materials and textures are a nod to the floral pattern behind the bed.

THIS DESK AREA could be an ordinary place, but the style gives real insight to Kayla's personality by showcasing favorite mementos.

THE FABRIC AND FRAME of a hand-me-down wing-back chair were updated with fresh coats of acrylic paint.

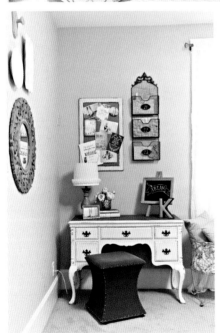

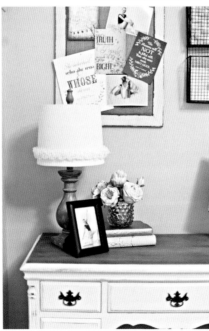

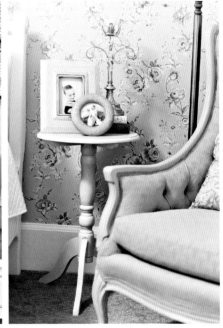

TYING IT TOGETHER

Elements of a Sanctuary

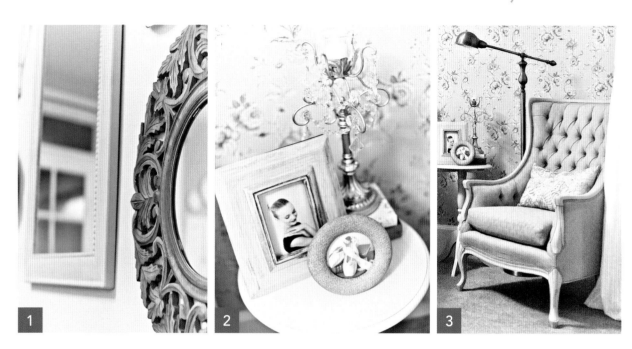

1   A VARIETY of shapes and sizes in this gallery wall adds an interesting mix of *details and materials*.

2   THINGS THAT MATTER, such as framed ballet photos, provide *inspiration* throughout Kayla's bedroom.

3   A REPURPOSED accent chair tucked into the corner next to a swing-arm floor lamp creates a *private space* for quiet contemplation.

Details and Materials

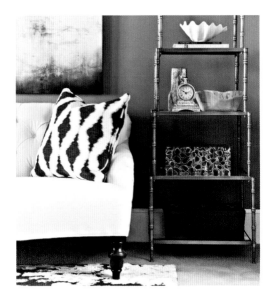

"The details are the details.
They make the design."

—Charles Eames

DETAILS AND MATERIALS

Attention to detail makes all the difference in the overall feel of a space. Whether those details are architectural or decorative, it's the little touch of something extra that expresses itself in a space.

Attention to detail is often what makes a space feel cohesive and complete whether we realize it or not. Details can be as minute as the style of a cabinet knob or as grand as wall of floor-to-ceiling windows. Details add character. The casing around a window, the shape of staircase, or the color of a ceiling all impact the overall feeling in a space.

Likewise, materials strongly influence our surroundings. The types of materials we choose, whether they are smooth, rough, soft, or hard are significant mood-setters. Materials affect our sense of sight and touch and can change the way a room feels—physically, mentally, emotionally, and spiritually. To keep a room from feeling sterile or too much of one set style, add a variety of texture and materials throughout.

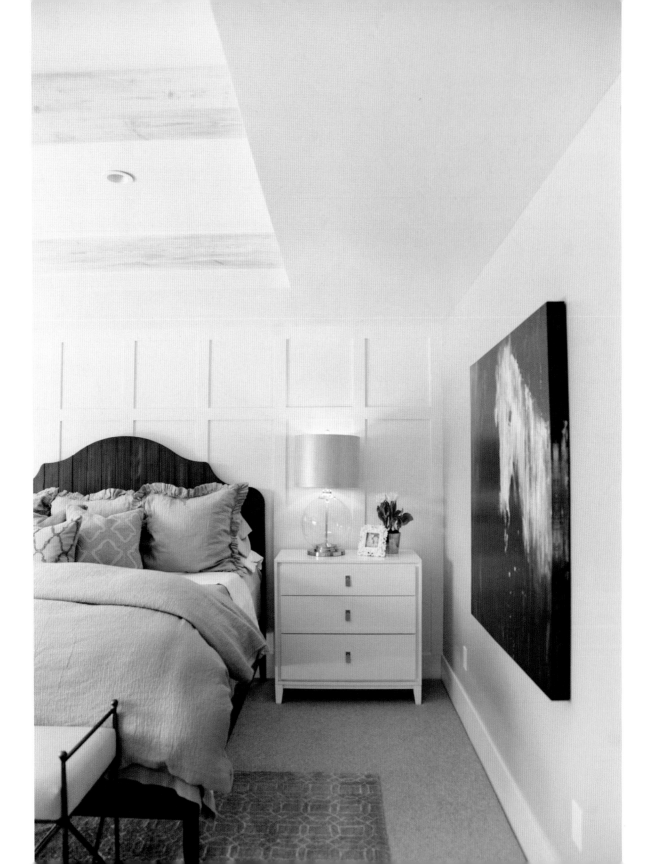

WIDE OPEN SPACE

One of the small luxuries Jeff and Tonya Olsen discovered in the 1960s rambler they purchased to remodel was the extraordinary size of the master bedroom. Bedrooms in homes from that era were typically small and efficient. The generous space allowed the Olsens to take creative liberty by adding a massive king-sized bed, chests of drawers as nightstands, and additional seating throughout.

The ceiling was coffered during the remodel, and Tonya added faux box beams to accentuate the refreshing detail. White-on-white board-and-batten was added to the wall behind the bed to further add subtle detailing. The wall treatment adds interest without overwhelming the room.

Tonya chose a neutral color palette for the space to purposely contrast the dramatic walnut platform bed and oversized headboard. She added dark accents throughout the room to tie it all together. The combination of contrasting materials gives the room a leisurely yet sophisticated feel.

Large-scale sliding doors were added to the south wall, expanding the space and flooding the room with light. The impressive view of the canyon and the valley below infuses the room with life.

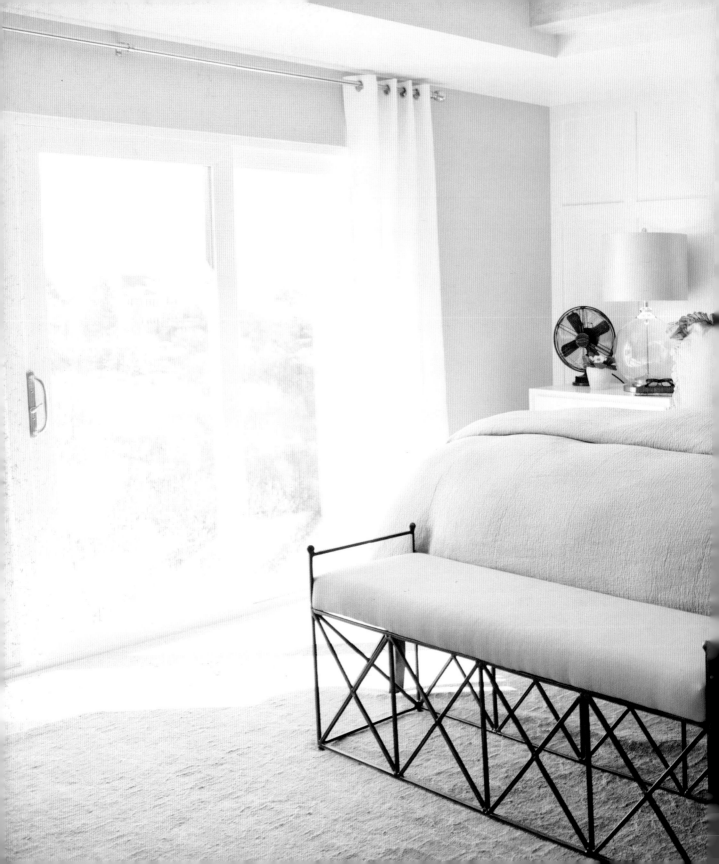

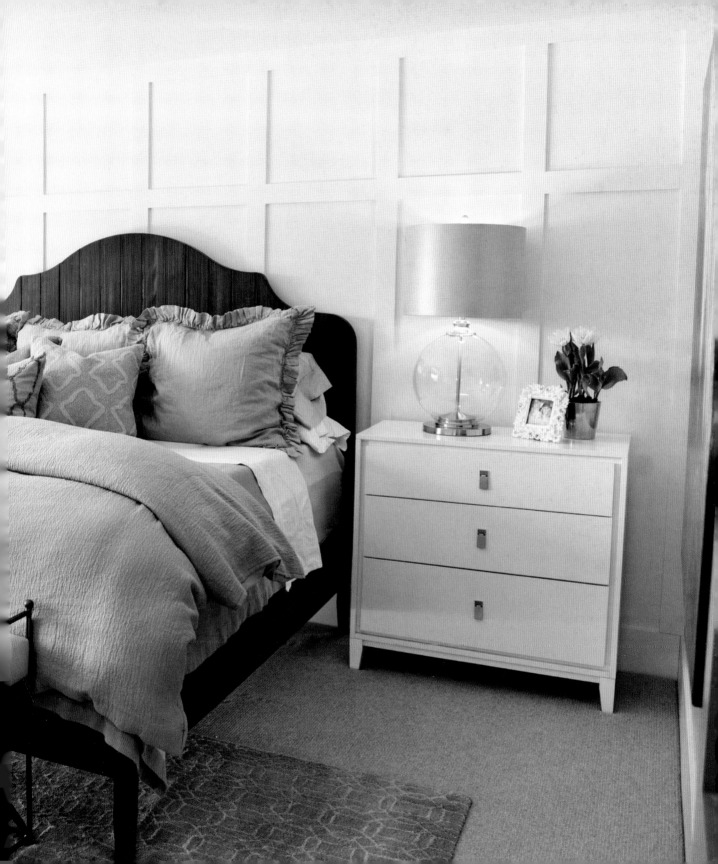

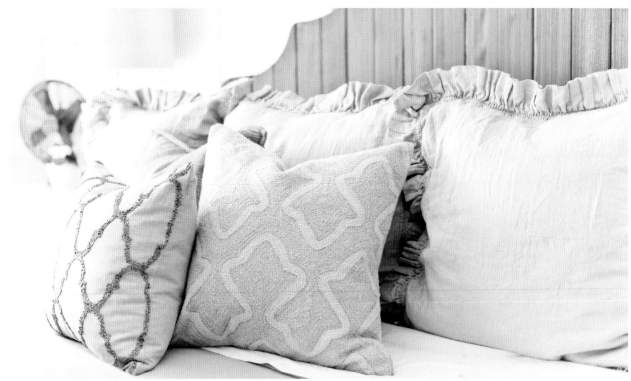

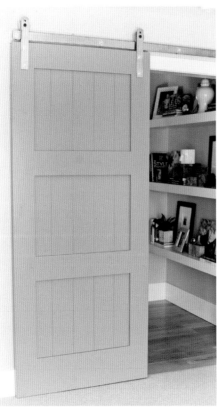
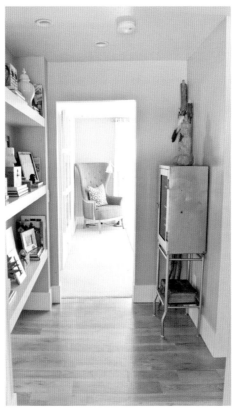

RICH AND DIVERSE materials adorn the bed, including organic cotton pillow shams, crisp white sheets, a flannel coverlet, and a grouping of beaded throw pillows.

A SLIDING BARN DOOR replaces the traditional door, adding another interesting detail and material to the space.

BUILT-IN SHELVING and a vintage medicine cabinet showcase treasured items directly outside the master bedroom door, leaving the bedroom itself free from distraction.

TYING IT TOGETHER

Elements of a Sanctuary

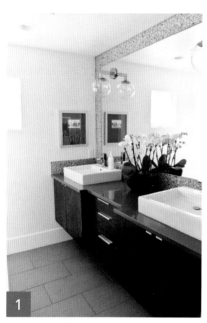
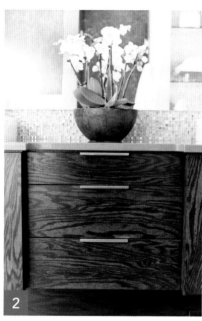
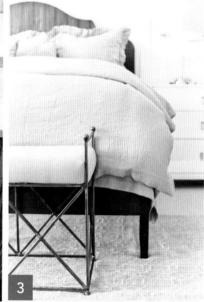

1   THE MASTER BATH, technically an extension of the master bedroom, is full of unique *details and materials*, including floating cabinets, 12 × 24-inch porcelain tile, and square vessel sinks.

2   THE CABINETS are built from quartersawn oak and stained a dark *color* that enhances the wood grain.

3   BILLOWY LINENS and a subtle color palette make this a perfect space for *meditation* and *prayer*.

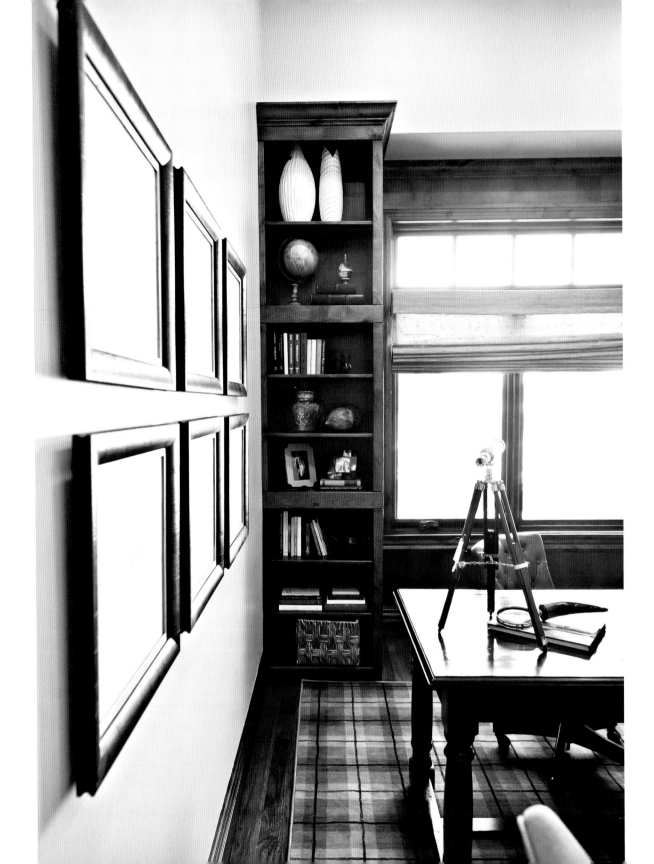

DOWN TO THE LAST DETAIL

Rachelle Olsen wanted the interior wood trim of her windows to really stand out in her new home. She knew designer Pamela Jensen would know exactly how to do that. Pamela designed open storage towers to add dimension and to frame the recessed windows.

Adjoining the entryway, a distinguished study full of warm woods, contemporary plaids, and masculine furniture serves as a secluded workspace for Rachelle's husband, Kyle. Another of Rachelle's favorite features is the stone arch in her entryway. To make the space feel traditional rather than rustic, Pamela suggested installing crisp white board-and-batten to the adjacent walls. The result is a stunning juxtaposition of textured and tailored finishes.

The combination of natural elements and classic details make this dream home worth coming back to.

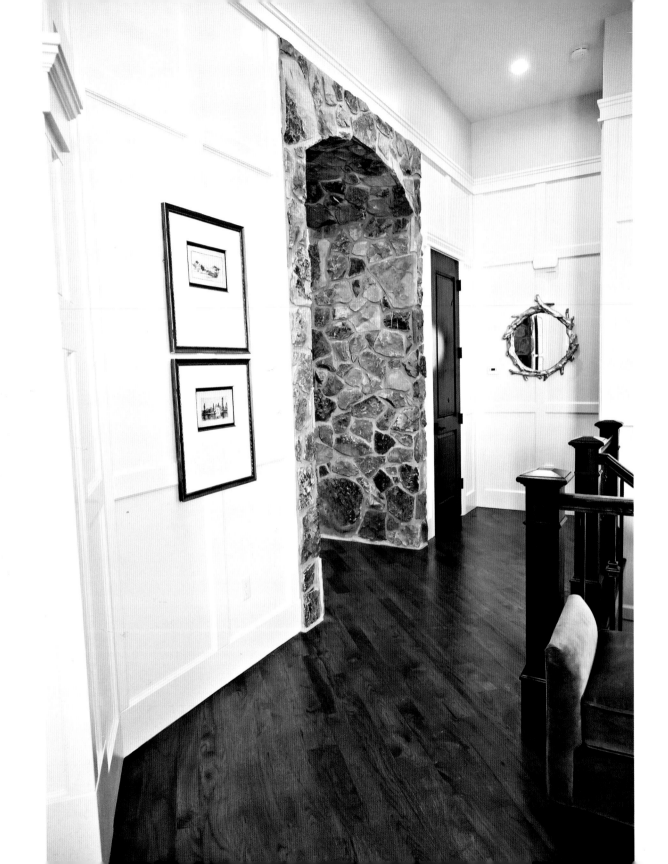

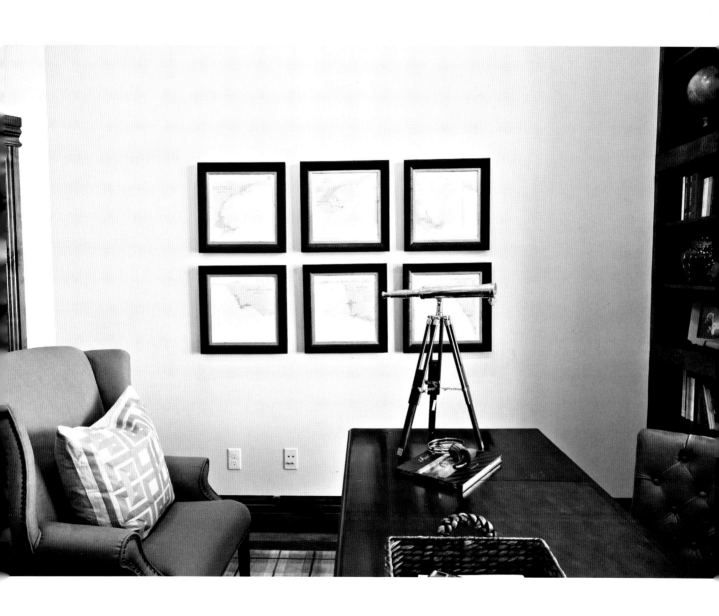

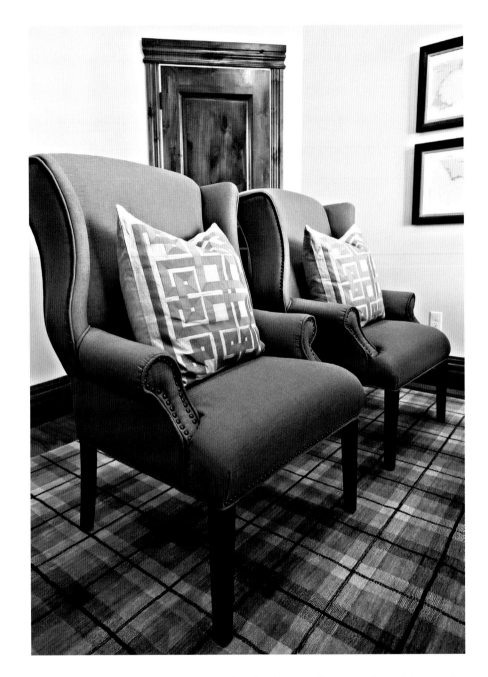

CLASSIC YET MASCULINE wing-back chairs offer comfortable seating for guests in the study. An exaggerated plaid rug anchors the space.

TYING IT TOGETHER

Elements of a Sanctuary

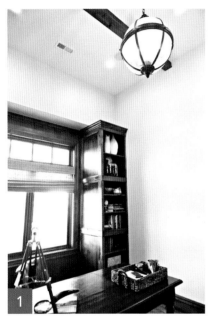 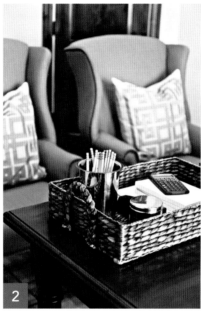 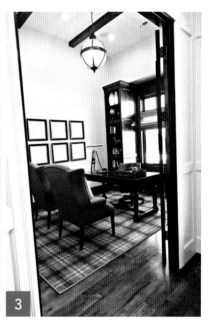

1   INTRICATE METALWORK details a traditional globe pendant that reflects the classic style of the space and adds ambient *light* in the evening.

2   A WICKER BASKET adds a practical touch by keeping desk essentials in *order*.

3   A SET OF DOUBLE DOORS make up the study entrance and can be closed to create a *private space*.

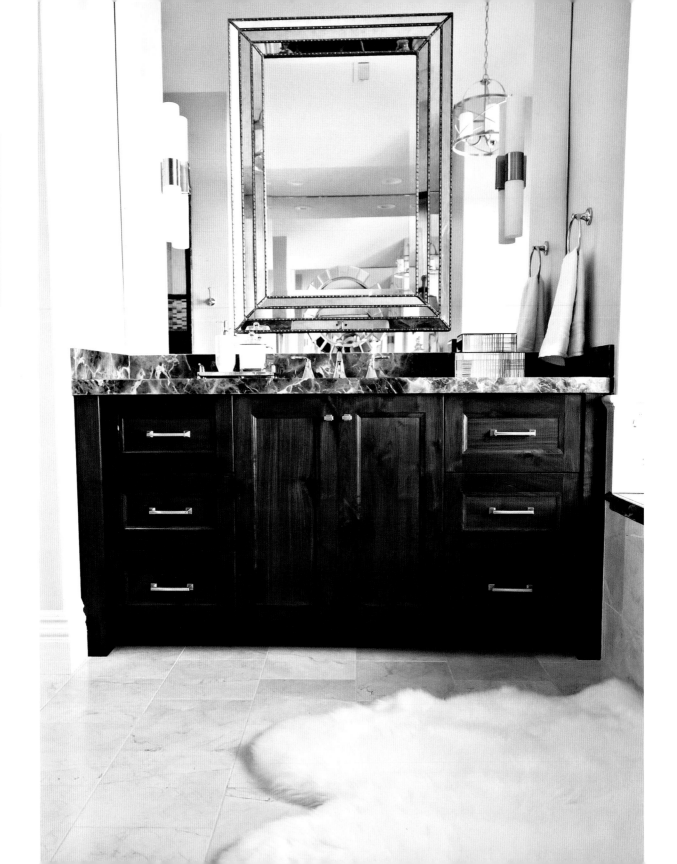

ESSENCE OF BEAUTY

A master bath should soothe mind, body, and spirit. That's exactly what designer Pamela Jensen helped create for Rachelle and Kyle Olsen in their new home.

A tongue and groove, barrel-vault ceiling highlights the entry into the opulent master bath. Ceramic, marble-styled tile inspires the soft neutral color scheme and the room's luxurious feeling. The eye-catching tile was installed in a brick pattern to add a touch of character. Functional linen curtain panels frame the window above the spacious soaking tub and add a soft feature to balance the solid surfaces throughout the room. Warm cabinetry and woodwork add to the timeless atmosphere. Finally, *his* and *hers* vanities, similarly designed yet individually unique, offer separate storage for Rachelle and Kyle.

An open floor plan combined with resplendent details make this master bath a peaceful getaway for the Olsens to enjoy.

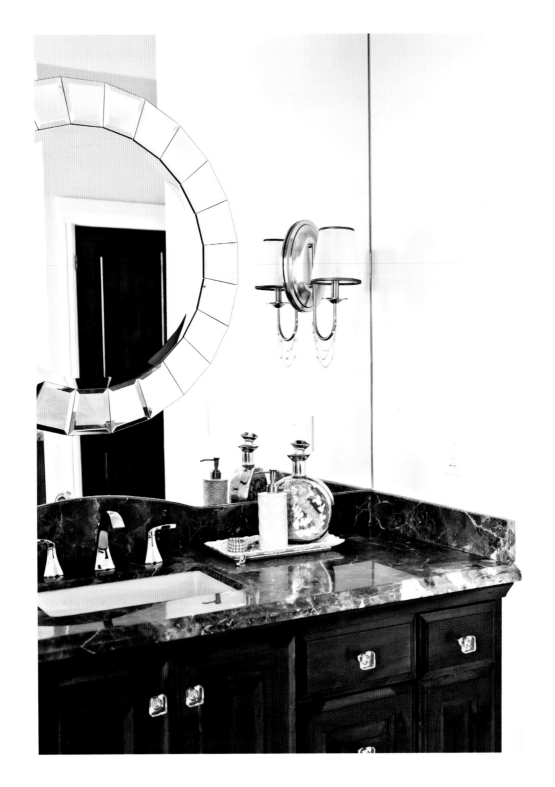

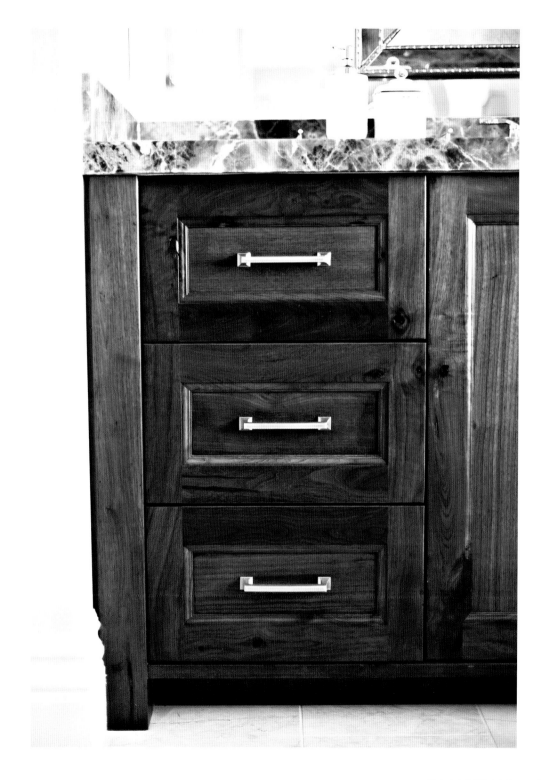

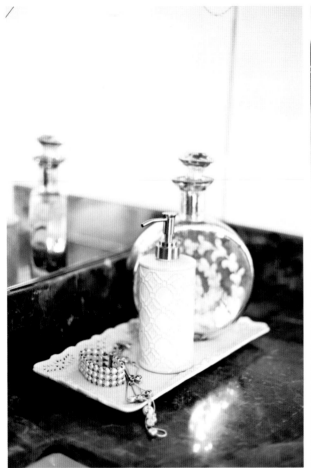
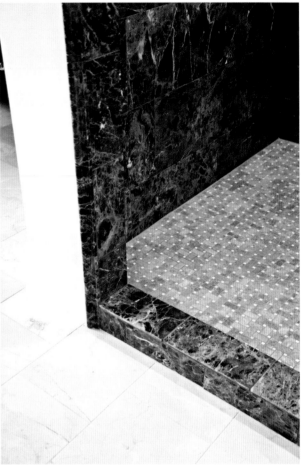

A PRETTY SERVING TRAY with lace detailing is used to hold dispensers, jars, and jewelry.

AN ITALIAN MARBLE basket-weave mosaic offsets the Emerpador dark marble surround in the master shower, creating a striking contrast.

TYING IT TOGETHER

Elements of a Sanctuary

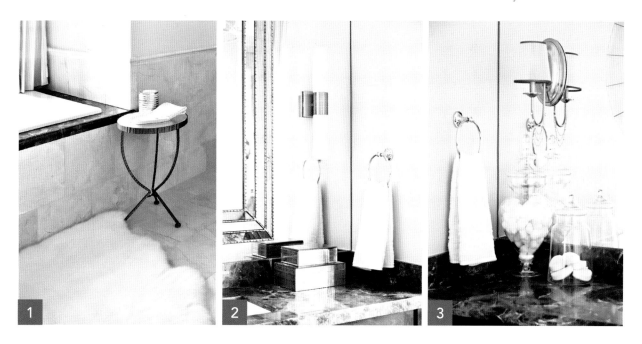

1   A COZY SHEEPSKIN RUG adds a soft and luxurious *detail* to the space.

2   A BEVELED MIRROR, conical sconces, and etched storage boxes add masculine *personality* to Kyle's vanity.

3   DELICATE GLASS apothecary jars keep soaps and cotton balls in *order*.

Things That Matter

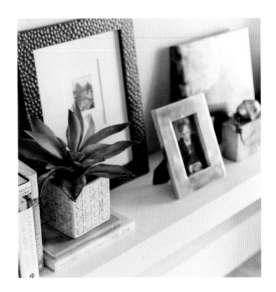

"Collect things you love, that are authentic to you, and your house becomes your story."

—Erin Flett

THINGS THAT MATTER

Showcasing things that matter, such as personal mementos, family photographs, and favorite objects, is one of the most meaningful ways of self-expression. Displaying our treasures makes a bold statement of who we are. Attractive displays and meaningful groupings are the best way to highlight things that matter. Special mementos conjure memories and can sometimes help get us through tough times.

A gallery wall of artwork, photographs, and objects is one of the easiest and most obvious forms of sharing things that matter. Mixing items of various sizes, colors, and shapes creates a work of art within itself. Conversely, hanging items in a symmetrical or linear layout creates a sense of balance and unity.

Propping things that matter on wall shelves is another way to express personality. Items that aren't permanently affixed to the wall allow for easy updates as our homes evolve over time. Varying shelf heights adds interest, while varying the quantity of items on display from shelf to shelf creates asymmetrical harmony. Grouping important objects of similar interest also maximizes impact.

The most powerful way to showcase things that matter is to surround yourself with the items you love and that inspire you.

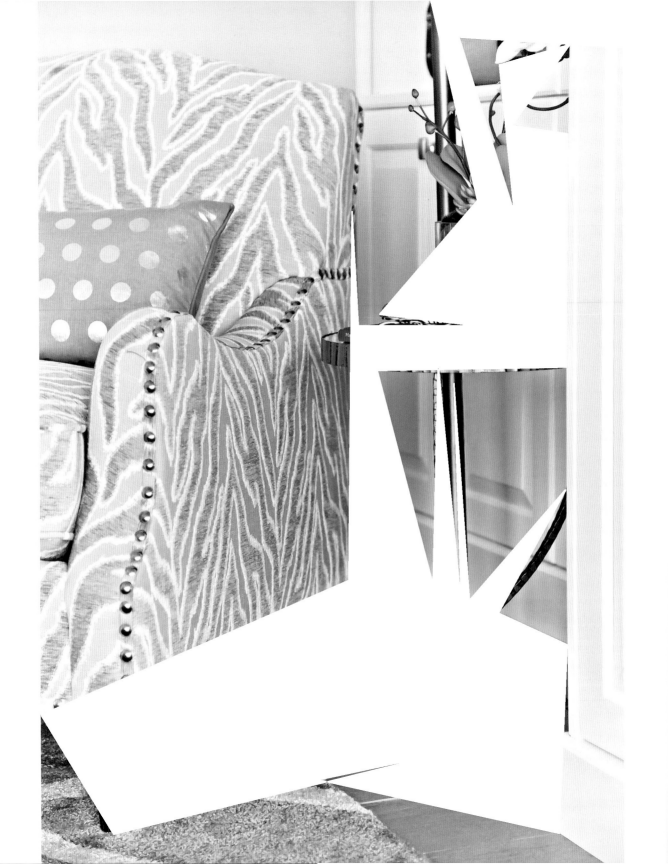

A FEW OF HER FAVORITE THINGS

Recently retired Laurie Riedinger moved from a charming bungalow in southern California to her custom-designed dream home surrounded by majestic mountains in northern Utah. The expansive size of her new home has plenty of room to showcase her collection of books, inherited treasures, and original artwork.

Laurie designed the home with plenty of open shelving for this purpose. Wall-to-wall shelves flank the fireplace in the family room. The open floor plan allows the *objets d'art* to be viewed from the kitchen area as well.

Designer Tonya Olsen assisted Laurie in arranging the space to highlight her vast assortment of collectibles. A comfy, oversized sectional is anchored by a generous area rug, creating a gathering space for friends and family to hang out in. Decorative accent chairs, including an oversized club chair covered in tone-on-tone zebra-striped fabric, are tucked in front of the bookshelves. This arrangement provides a comfortable place for reading with easy access to the library of books.

The walls were painted Laurie's favorite color, turquoise. The beachy color lends a southern-California vibe while contrasting the crisp white cabinets and finish work throughout the home.

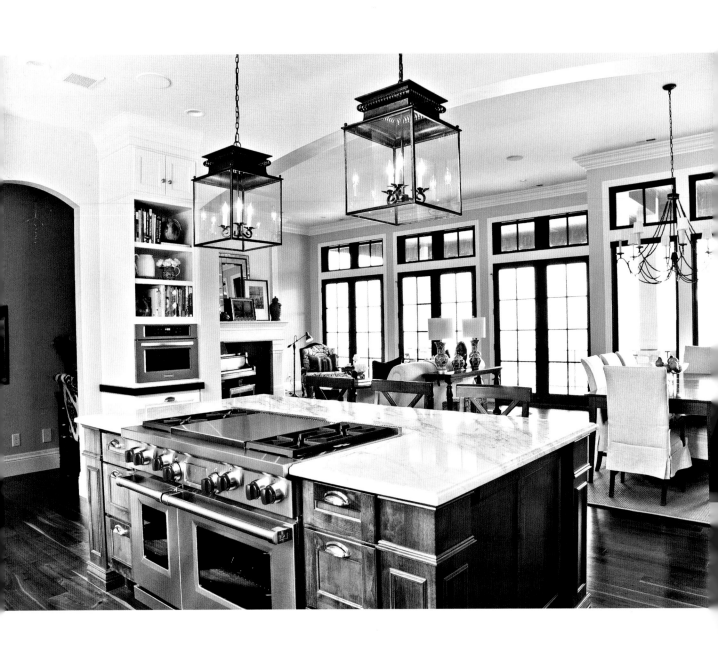

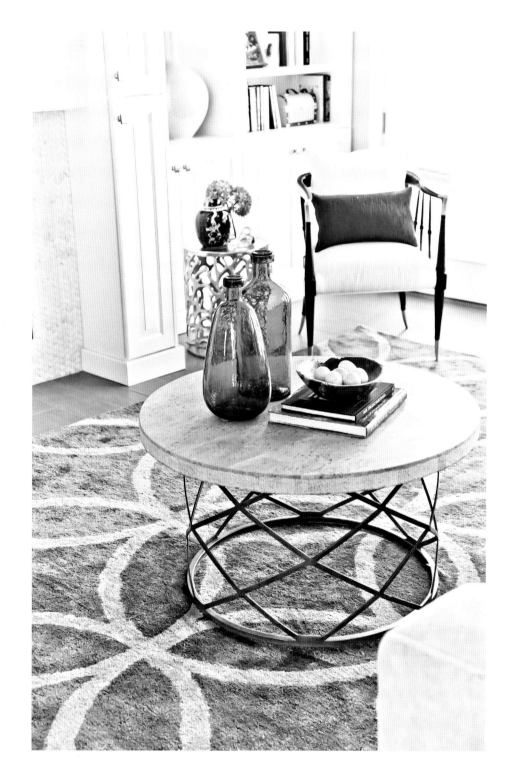

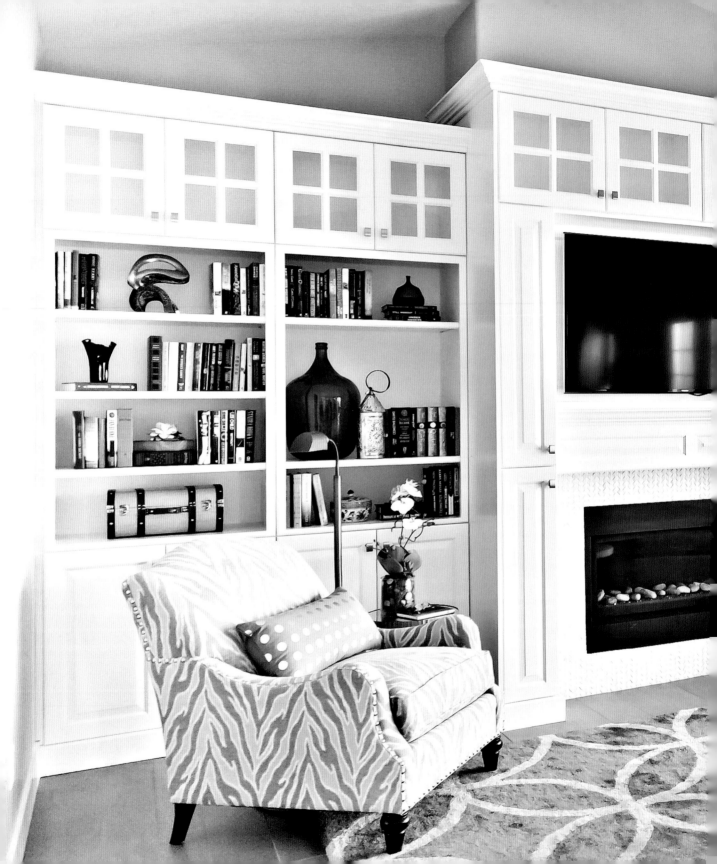

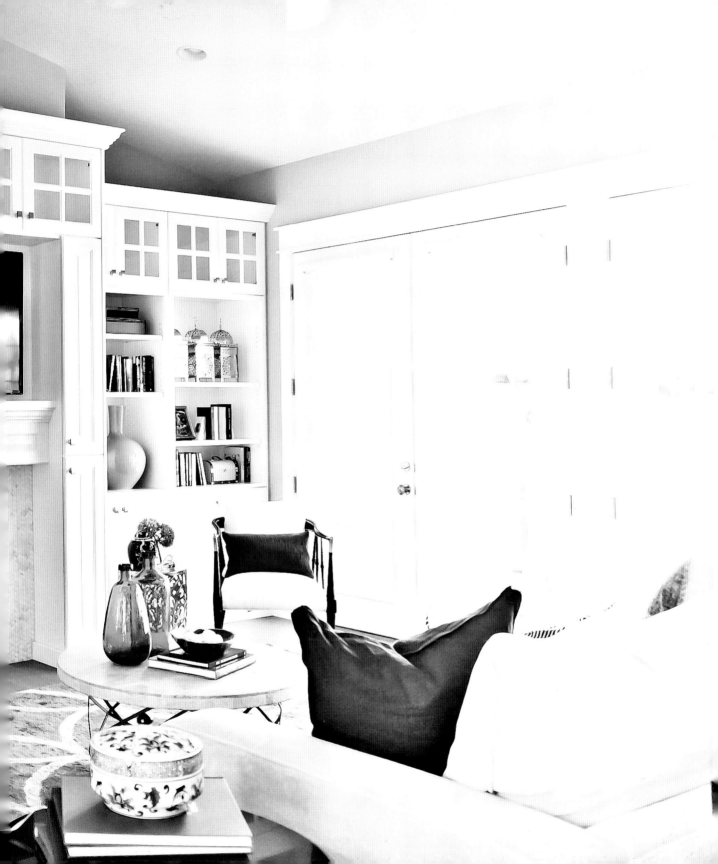

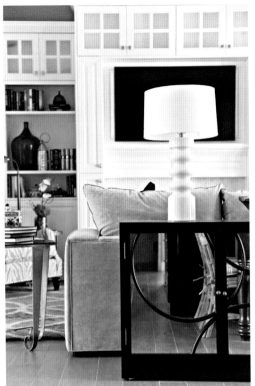

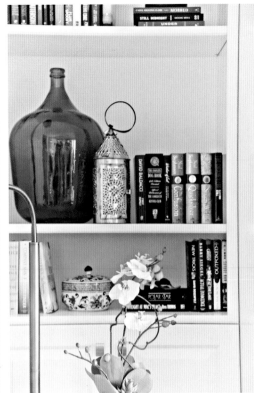

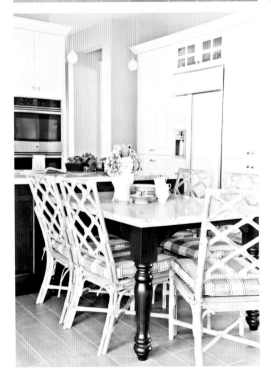

A CONSOLE table with mirrored doors is used behind the sectional as storage for additional keepsakes that might not be as attractive to display.

LAYERED GROUPINGS of treasures interspersed among stacks and rows of books add depth and interest to the space.

AN ATTACHED dining table extrudes from the island to create a cohesive flow from the kitchen to the family room. Bamboo dining chairs add a touch of southern-California character.

TYING IT TOGETHER

Elements of a Sanctuary

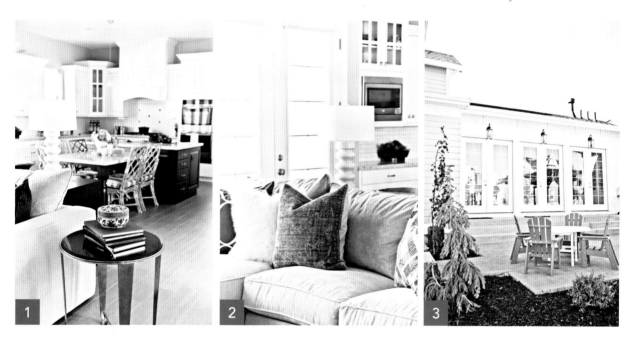

1   AN OPEN FLOOR PLAN includes casual dining and combines with the adjoining family room to create a large, open *gathering space*.

2   ACCENT LIGHTING is found in both the family room and kitchen to introduce plenty of *lighting* options for various tasks.

3   FRENCH DOORS drench the interior with natural light and connect the space to *nature*. When the doors are open, the family room is connected with an adjacent patio.

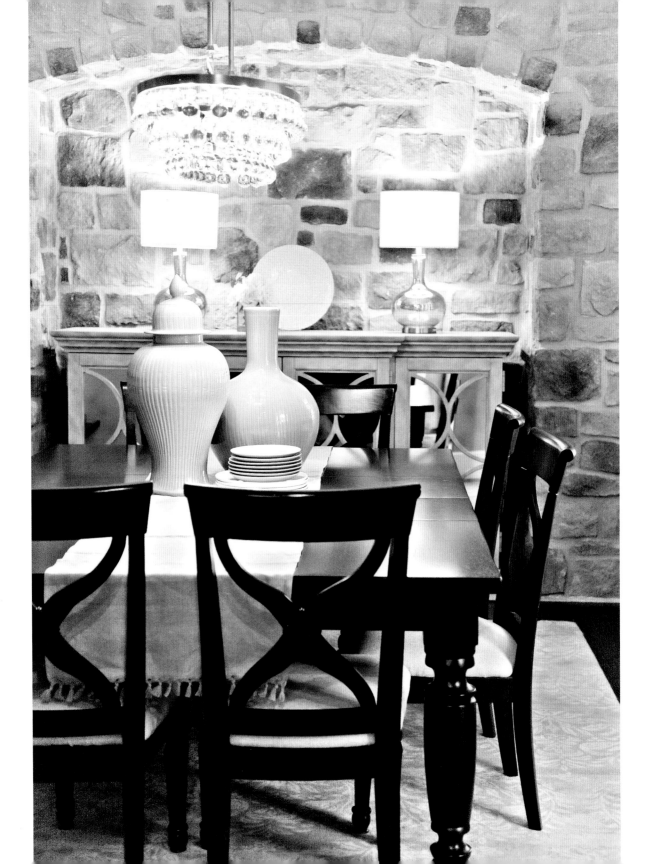

SET IN STONE

Kristy Feller's dining room served its purpose. Sure, the dining set provided plenty of seating for her family of six, but the uninspired room lacked character and personality. Kristy enlisted the help of designer Deboni Sacre to take the much-used, functional space from mundane to magnificent.

An arched stone niche provided an interesting architectural detail in the space. Since Kristy wanted to add a spot for storage, it turned out to be the quintessential spot to place a serving buffet. The closed-door cabinet stores extra dinnerware, serving plates, and linens. A set of matching mercury table lamps illuminates the recessed alcove and provides ambient lighting in the room.

A decorative glass chandelier adds sparkle to the space. Wall-to-wall shelves showcase the family's collection of artwork and can be appreciated when the family gathers for meals.

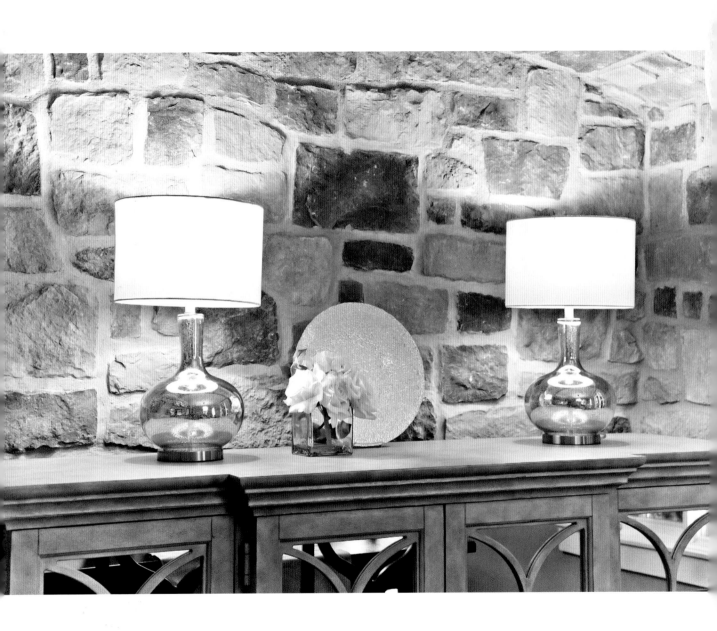

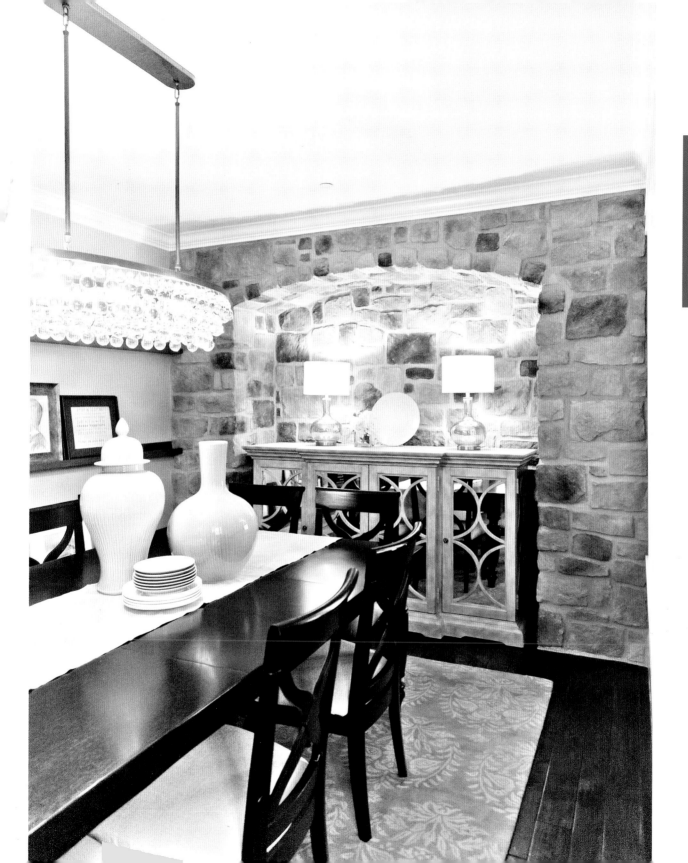

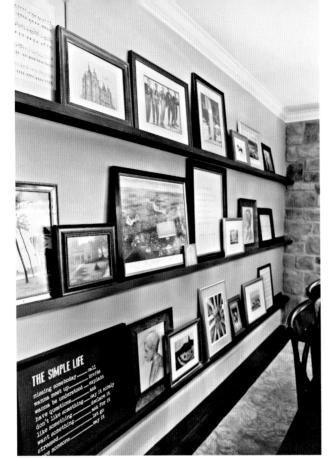

A CASUAL MIX of things that matter lines the dining room wall, while a crystal chandelier adds a glamorous touch to the eclectic space.

INSTEAD OF HANGING artwork in a traditional gallery format, wall-length wooden shelves were installed for propping and layering an assortment of framed artwork, sketches, music, and portraits, creating a dramatic focal point in the space.

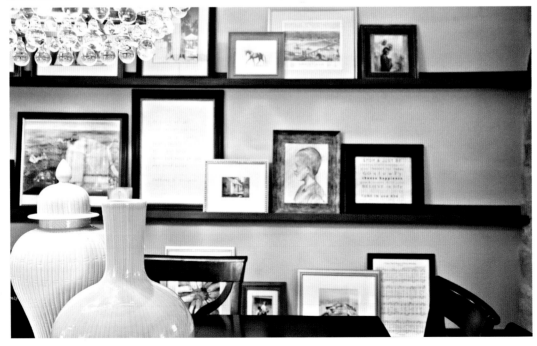

TYING IT TOGETHER

Elements of a Sanctuary

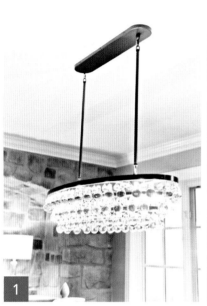
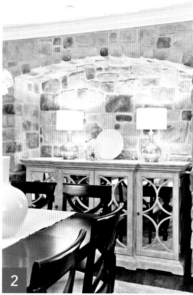
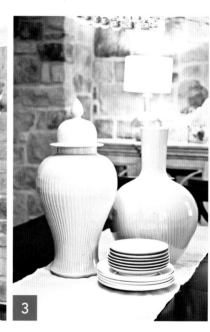

1 AN ELEGANT CHANDELIER, mercury table lamps, and natural *lighting* illuminate the space and offer a variety of combinations for creating ambience.

2 A MIRRORED BUFFET is nestled into a stone niche. The size of the cabinet is a perfect example of the design principles of *scale and proportion*.

3 WHILE THE VALUES RANGE from dark to light throughout the room, a touch of *color* using decorative jars in a subtle mid-tone keeps the room from feeling too stark.

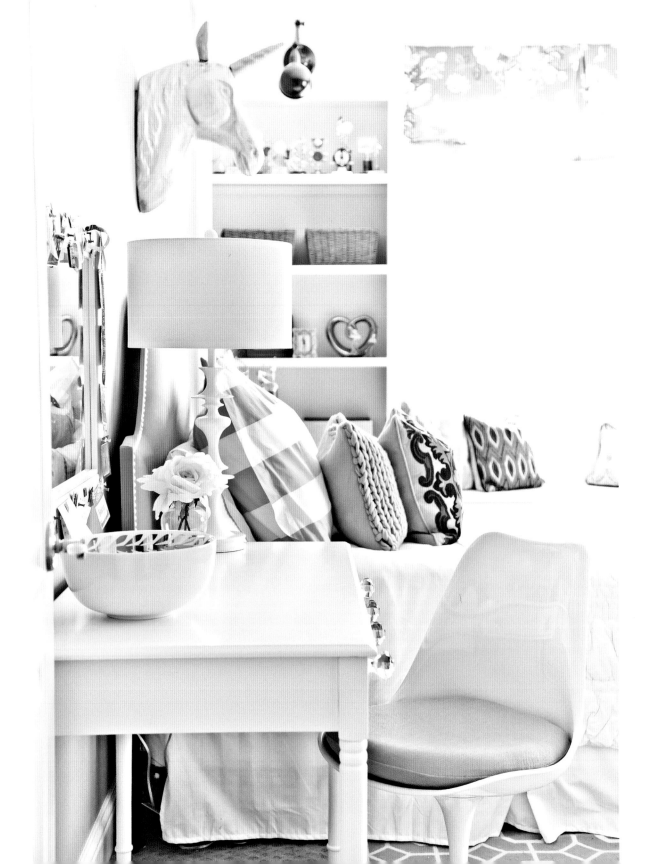

ROOM TO GROW

While working on the bedroom design for lighthearted teen Brooklyn Baldwin, designer Pamela Jensen often joked with her that it was one of the most expensive projects she had ever worked on. They were working on a limited budget to design the room, but Brooklyn's impressive collection of dance pictures, competition trophies, and one-of-a-kind snow globes from around the world surely cost her mom a pretty penny.

With such a grand quantity of personal mementos, Pamela wanted to make sure the room properly showcased Brooklyn's collections.

Brooklyn first and foremost wanted her room to be an expression of herself. Pamela installed shelves, making it easy for Brooklyn to display her treasures while easily trading them out over time. As she gathers new mementos, she can simply replace an existing one, keeping her room updated and relevant.

The color palette was inspired by one of Brooklyn's favorite floral fabrics. The white foundation makes the room feel fresh and bright while the pops of turquoise, pink, and apple green add a vibrant touch.

To finish the design, Pamela hung a metallic unicorn head above Brooklyn's custom coral headboard. The result is a whimsical space that Brooklyn can call her own.

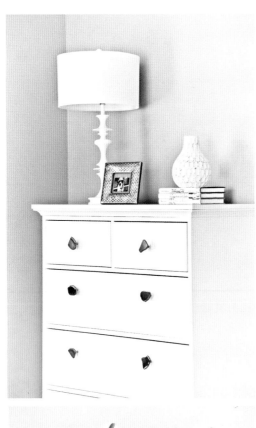

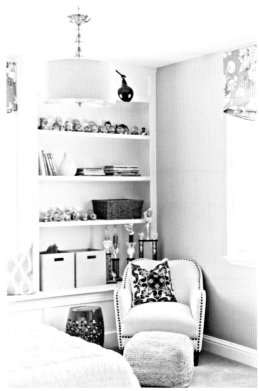

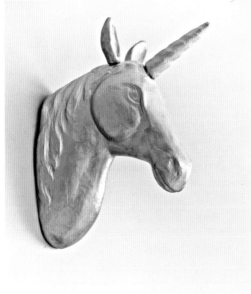

AN INEXPENSIVE dresser is personalized with an assortment of funky decorative hardware.

CUSTOM BUILT-INS not only house all of Brooklyn's things that matter but they also add a seating and storage element.

WHAT TEENAGE GIRL'S bedroom is complete without a metallic unicorn head? The eccentric accessory reflects Brooklyn's whimsical personality.

TYING IT TOGETHER

Elements of a Sanctuary

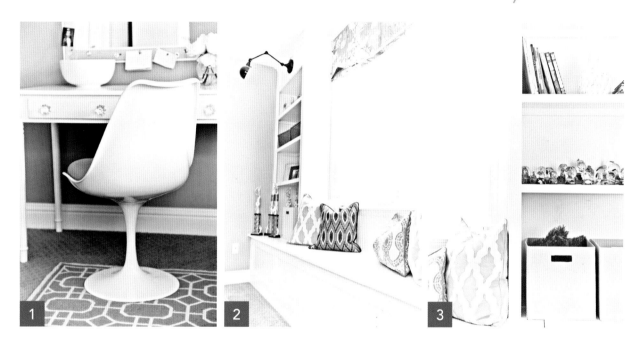

1 THIS TEEN BEDROOM is bursting with *personality*. In addition to the bright colors and personal collections, a replicate Eero Saarinen Tulip chair adds a modern touch to the space.

2 BROOKLYN'S BEDROOM doubles as a *gathering space* for friends to hang out in. A bench seat, desk chair, and pouf provide extra seating.

3 STORAGE IS IMPORTANT to keep a teen bedroom in *order*. Fabric baskets provide concealed storage, and open shelving works as a decorative display.

Reflection

REFLECTION

Sacred geometry is the belief that numbers and patterns, such as the divine ratio, have sacred significance. Many mystical and spiritual practices, including astrology, numerology, tarot, and feng shui, begin with a fundamental belief in sacred geometry. Architects and designers may draw upon concepts of sacred geometry when they choose particular geometric forms to create pleasing, soul-satisfying spaces.

A spiritual atmosphere is a calm, peaceful atmosphere and is equally as essential to our well-being as the mental, emotional, and physical. In today's hurried world, places for meditation, where we can slow down and focus on what really matters, are fewer and fewer.

A home is a place for nurturing and teaching the next generation. In the home, we create moments and places to teach family members both secular and spiritual lessons, including values and moral and ethical standards.

A spiritual atmosphere has low-contrast colors that soothe the soul and allow for meditation. Creating a spiritual atmosphere whether at a church, synagogue, temple, or at home has much to do with the lighting. Chandeliers sparkle and give off an ethereal or heavenly feeling. Warm, natural sunlight streaming into a room can instantly create a spiritual feeling. A spiritual atmosphere needn't be in every room of the home, but it should be in key rooms where you want to create spiritual moments.

Interior Reflection

ASK YOURSELF THE FOLLOWING QUESTIONS WHEN CONTEMPLATING
THE SPIRITUAL ATMOSPHERE OF YOUR HOME:

1. Does my decor reflect a spiritual environment conducive to meditation?
2. Are the colors in my space soft and subtle?
3. How can I incorporate spiritual symbolism that is important to me into my space?
4. Is my space quiet? Private?
5. How is nature infused into my spiritual space?

Inspiration and Symbolism

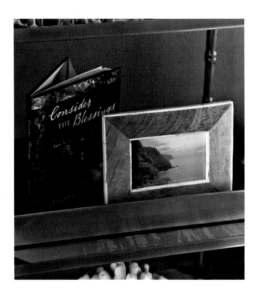

"Good design has to tell a story. It has to stop people, and it has to make them wonder."

—Zahid Sardar

INSPIRATION AND SYMBOLISM

Symbols are everywhere. They can be found in history, nature, business, and especially in our homes. While some are more understandable than others, we intuitively know the instant we see a symbol if we understand its meaning. Experts that study the effects of design psychology believe that the symbols within our surroundings have a fundamental effect on our physical, mental, emotional, and spiritual well-being. The items we choose for our homes, whether consciously or subconsciously, tend to resonate with symbolic meaning.

Inspirational items have symbolic meanings as well. Photos of our family heritage, motivational books and music, and artwork are simple yet profound accents we can incorporate into our homes. Surrounding ourselves with these personal items greatly influences our well-being whether we realize it or not.

The psychology of color has a profound impact on your instantaneous reaction to color. Colors have many layers of significance and symbolic associations. For example, the color red is often associated with intensity, love, and danger. When incorporating specific colors in your home, be conscious of how those colors resonate with you personally.

Like color, shapes also have symbolic meaning. The meaning behind a certain shape is influenced culturally, personally, and contextually by its surroundings. Squares represent and suggest order, stability, and security; circles, on the other hand, represent unity, wholeness, and perfection.

The colors we choose and the style of furniture and decor in our homes has a significant symbolic effect on us. When designing your sanctuary, be aware of how these symbols play a role in your environment.

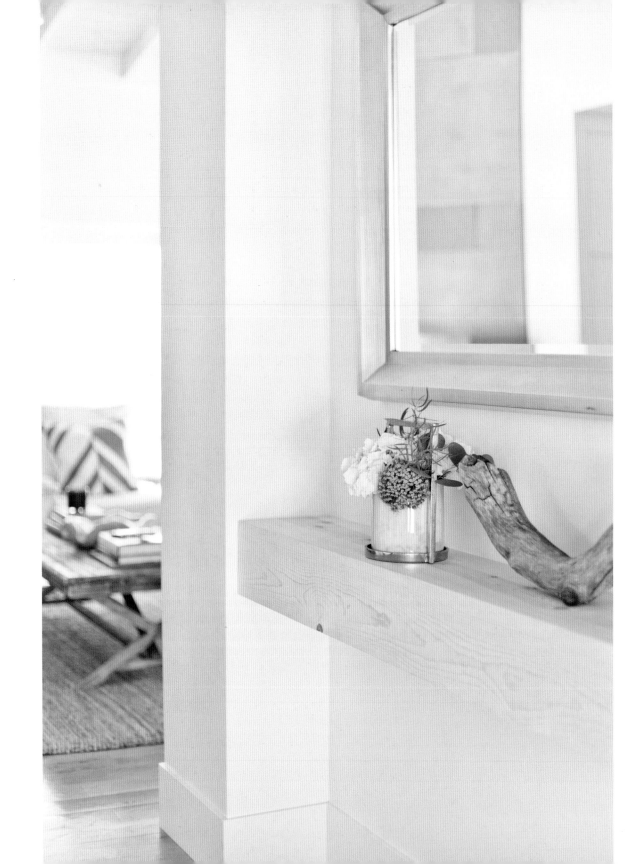

MAKE AN ENTRANCE

An inviting entryway sets the tone for the rest of a home and should be designed around the hustle and bustle of coming and going. Sometimes, though, this space is overlooked and often lacks a thoughtful design approach.

Jeff and Tonya Olsen wanted their entry to immediately convey an essence of who they are and what they represent as a family. Jeff's love of sacred geometry is apparent in the meaningful symbols incorporated into the architectural and decorative design of the space.

For starters, the set of languid blue-green double doors represents balance, peace, growth, and harmony. Semiopaque decorative glass allows natural light to softly illuminate the space while providing a modicum of privacy.

A six-foot square entry rug grounds the symmetrical space. Historically, a square represents balance, grounding, and foundation, which convey a sense of stability upon entering the home. Directly above the area rug, a large entry light encased in a circular drum shade represents unity and wholeness.

Minimal decor and an oversized mirror complete the look of this interesting entryway and serve as a symbolic prelude the rest of the Olsens' home.

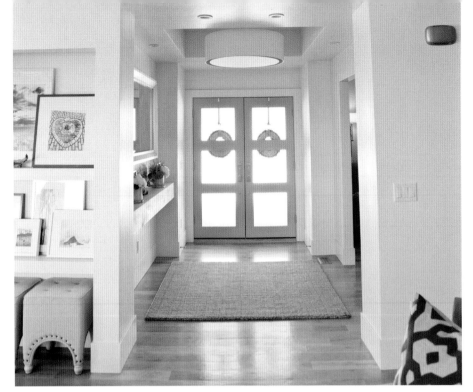

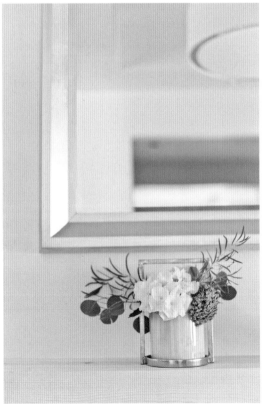

THE ENTRY was designed to be symmetrical and ingrained with symbolic shapes and meaning.

A SIMPLE flower arrangement greets visitors in the entry. White chrysanthemums picked fresh from the garden represent honesty.

TYING IT TOGETHER

Elements of a Sanctuary

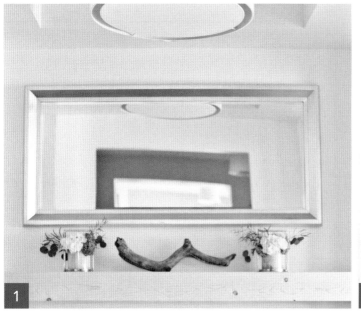

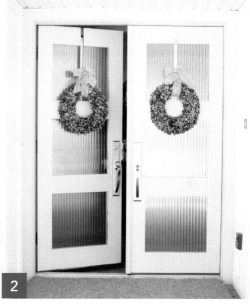

1   THE OVERSIZED entry mirror is a symbol of physical and spiritual *reflection*.

2   THE BLUE-GREEN COLOR of the entry doors represents balance. A set of ornamental green wreaths symbolically represents strength and add an element of *nature*.

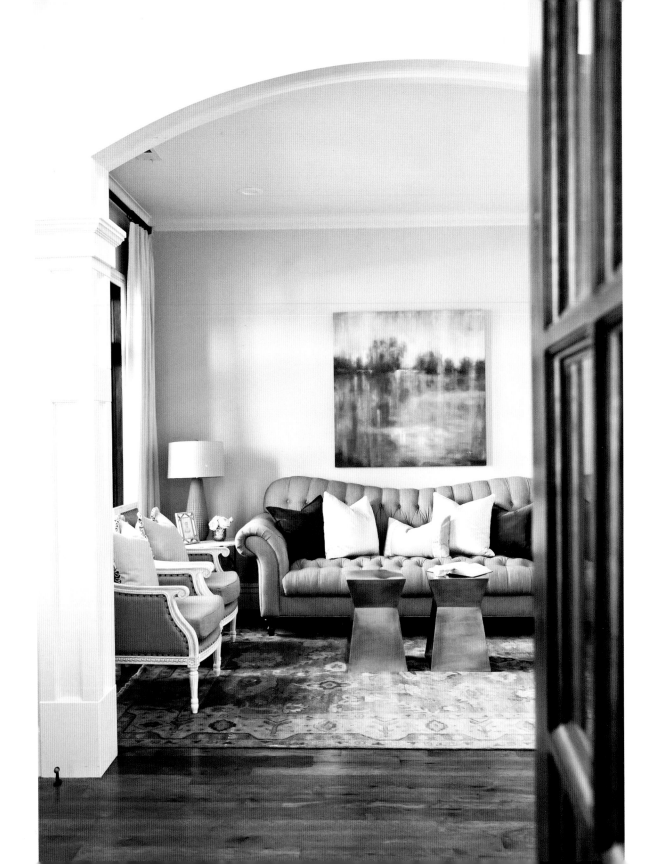

MUSICAL INSPIRATION

The sweet sound of the piano is often heard flowing through Rachelle Olsen's home from one of her four musically inclined children. Encouraged to begin lessons at age four, the Olsen children spend endless hours at the piano, so Rachelle wanted their music room to be a melodic source of inspiration.

Designer Pamela Olsen chose a soft color palette of blue, green, and gray to anchor the space and contrasted it with dramatic yet understated artwork. Billowy linen curtains frame the floor-to-ceiling windows, softening the overall feel of the space. Classically designed furniture creates an inviting conversation area for guests.

The combined result is a musical tapestry full of colorful and intricate design details.

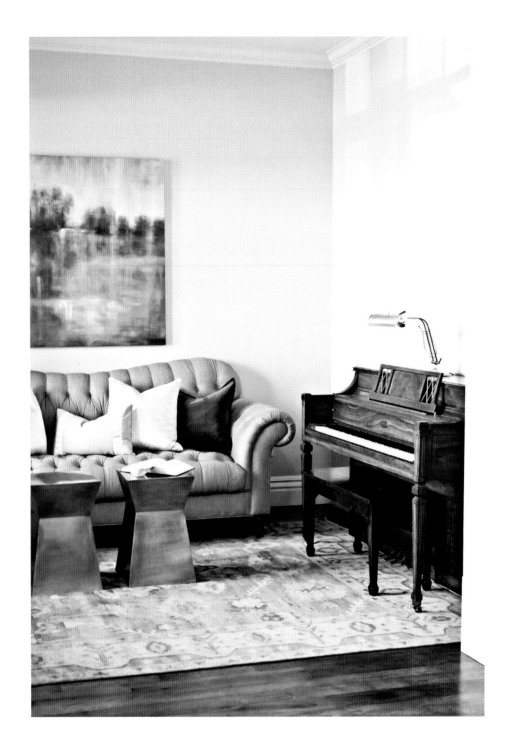

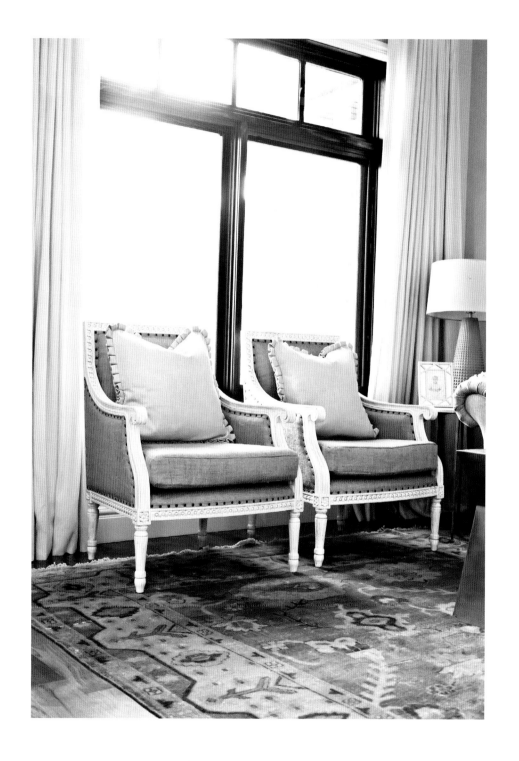

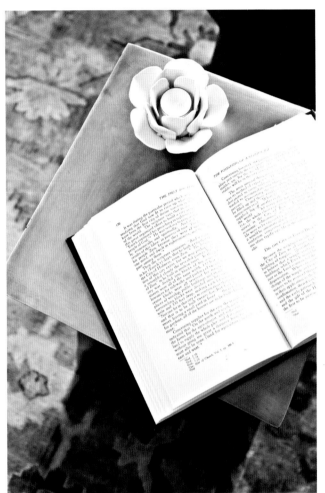

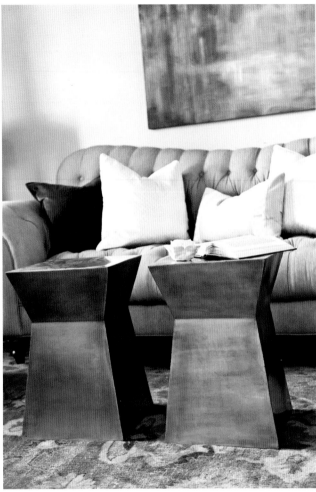

THE SERENE DECOR and solitude of this space makes it the perfect spot for enjoying an inspirational book.

SMALL PEDESTALS paired together serve as a coffee table or additional seating.

TYING IT TOGETHER

Elements of a Sanctuary

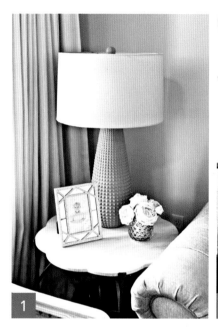
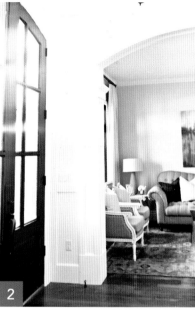
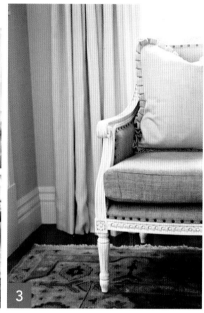

1 ACCENT LIGHTS, such as table lamps, provide a warm glow in the evening. Curtains can also be drawn to change the mood of the space.

2 ADDED DETAIL in the paneled woodwork makes the entrance to the sitting room more formal.

3 BURLAP UPHOLSTERED CHAIRS and linen drapery panels add an element of *nature* to the space.

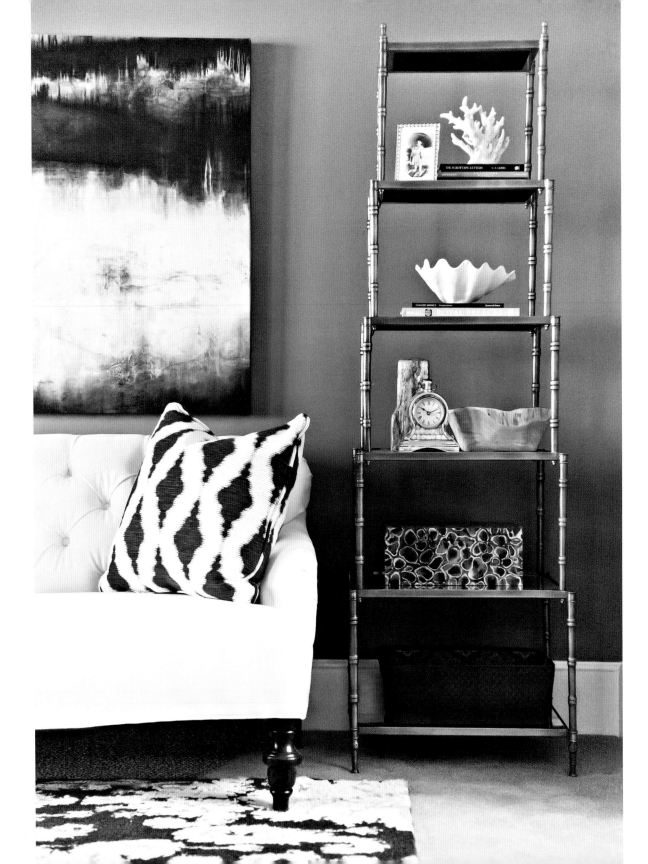

INSPIRED ELEGANCE

Historically, a parlor was a small private room adjacent to an entry for receiving guests. Few homes today have such a room, but Kristy Feller decided to change an unused room at the front of her home into exactly that. The first step was to move the family piano. This created an opportunity for the space to have new purpose. Kristy enlisted the help of designer Deboni Sacre to take the space in a new direction.

Deboni added two elegant *étagères* and an inspirational piece of artwork above the small-scale sofa. These simple additions immediately balanced the space. An area rug in moody hues anchors the space. Coordinating throw pillows and an assortment of favorite objects made the room complete.

Kristy requested that the room be filled with inspirational items as well. Photos of meaningful people, books, and music accessorize the space, igniting sparks of inspiration. Now, soft music plays in the background as the Fellers greet their guests and welcome them to their home in style.

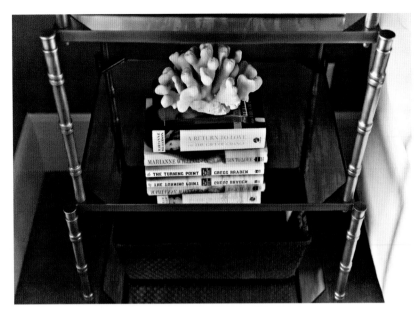

PERSONAL and inspiring items are layered on the one of the *étagères*, including a religious book and a favorite postcard.

INSPIRATIONAL, hardbound books are stacked as a pedestal for a favorite souvenir.

STRATEGICALLY PLACING items of inspiration in an easy-to-reach, convenient location is a great way to encourage guests to access them.

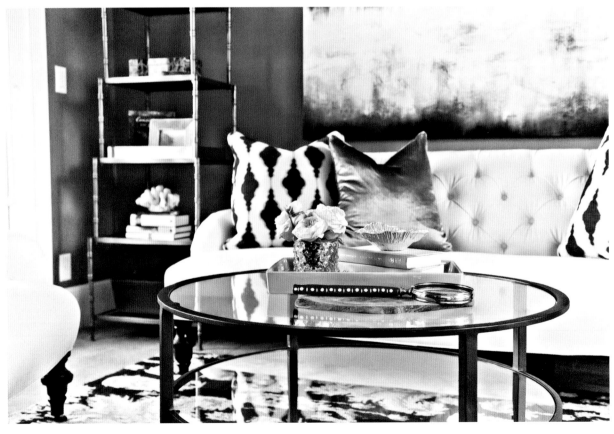

TYING IT TOGETHER

Elements of a Sanctuary

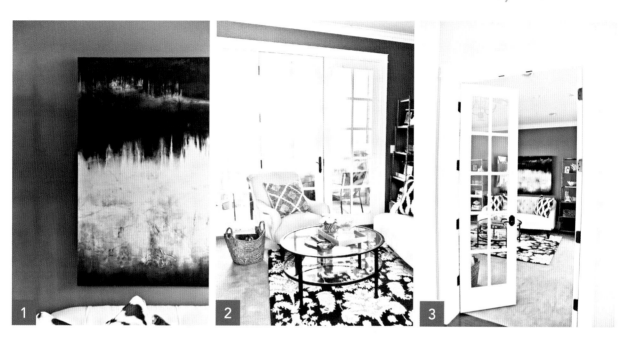

1   THE CAPRICIOUS ARTWORK, though dark and moody, lends the room to *meditation* and *reflection*.

2   A VIEW OF NATURE is warm and welcoming through a series of french doors.

3   FRENCH DOORS flank two sides of this room, allowing it to be open to the activity of the household or closed off as a *private space*.

Meditation and Reflection

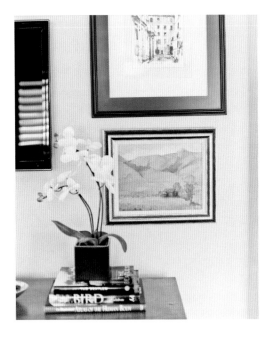

"A house is much more than a mere shelter;
it should lift us emotionally and spiritually."

—John Saladino

MEDITATION AND REFLECTION

A sanctuary used for personal reflection has an atmosphere of serenity and tranquility. Comfortable surroundings, understated furnishings, and simple decor are key for creating a personal space for meditation and prayer.

Designing a space conducive to personal reflection often requires using a natural color palette. Quiet, neutral colors, reflective of the earth and sky, instill a sense of calmness. Simple furnishings and uncluttered surfaces help to minimize distractions. It probably goes without saying that eliminating cell phones and televisions from such a space will further enhance a contemplative experience.

The scale and proportion of a room has an effect on the tranquility of a space. Quaintness gives a sense of coziness. Creating the right variations so the home feels comfortable will also help it feel like a sanctuary.

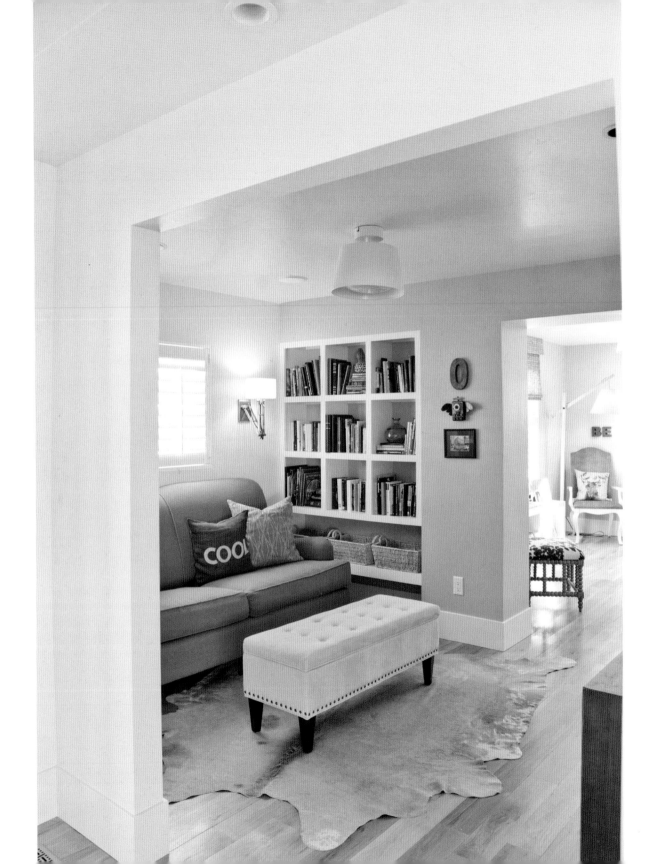

MULTIPURPOSE RETREAT

Tonya and her husband Jeff made a conscious decision to keep their television out of their main living room. Jeff was adamant that the living room was to be used as a conversation area and to be enjoyed for its sweeping views of the canyon and the dramatic stone fireplace. During their remodel, a location for the TV became a main concern. Ultimately, the Olsens chose to place it in an adjacent sitting room.

The TV is cleverly "hidden in plain sight" amongst a gallery wall of artwork. This gives the television its place of honor without making it the star of the room. A mid-century console given to Tonya as an anniversary gift provides plenty of storage for DVDs and components.

Built-in symmetrical shelving, stacked full with favorite books and mementos, bookend a comfy sofa. Wicker baskets house a collection of vintage records. Above the sofa, adjustable swing-arm wall lamps offer flexibility for reading. An upholstered ottoman provides a place for feet propping and storage for blankets. The cowhide rug, reminiscent of Jeff's days growing up on a farm, adds an eclectic touch to the space.

In addition to serving the family as a library and TV room, the multifunctional space is the perfect in-between space for meditation and reflection.

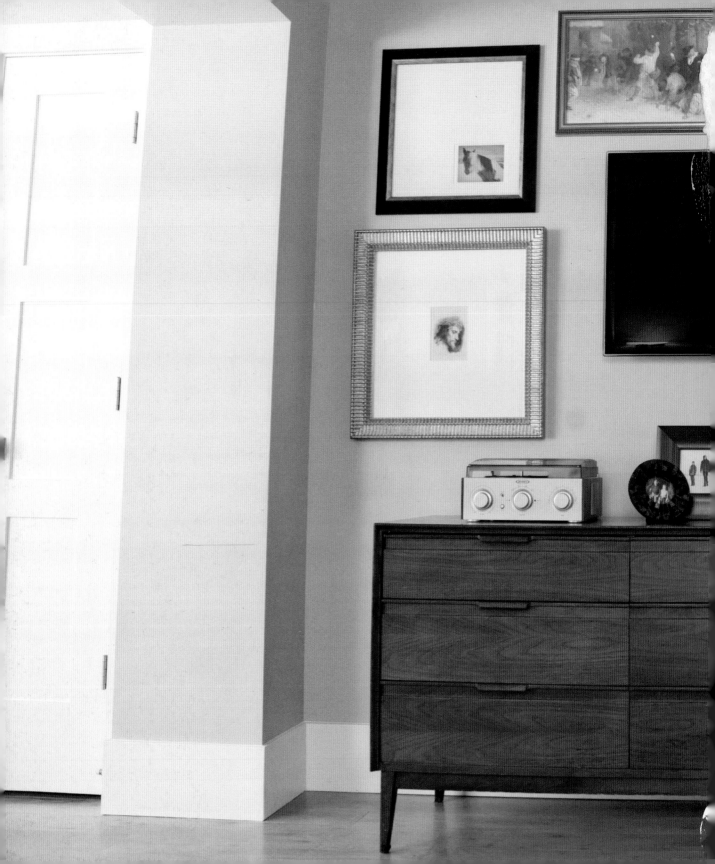

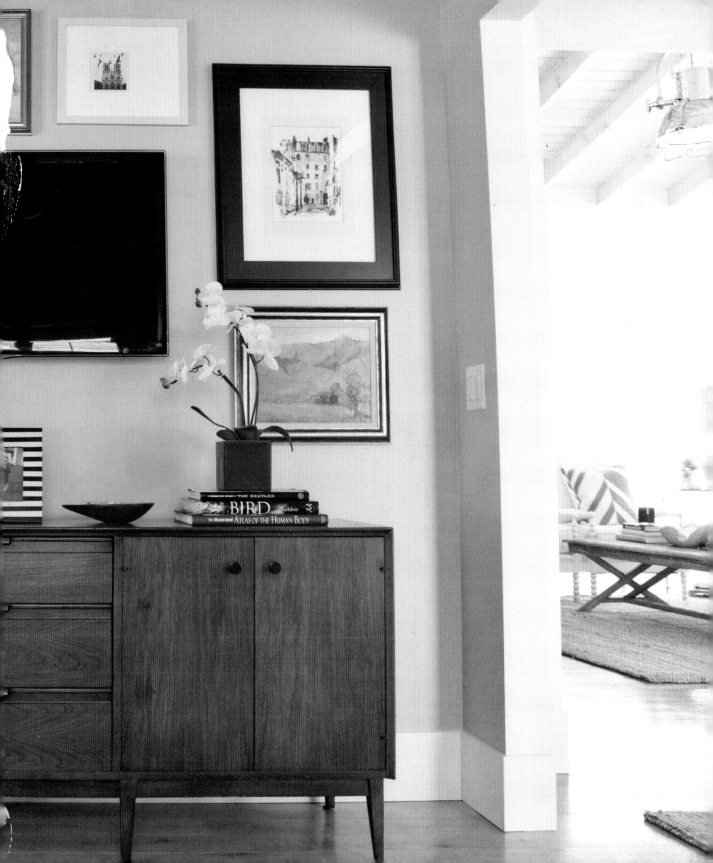

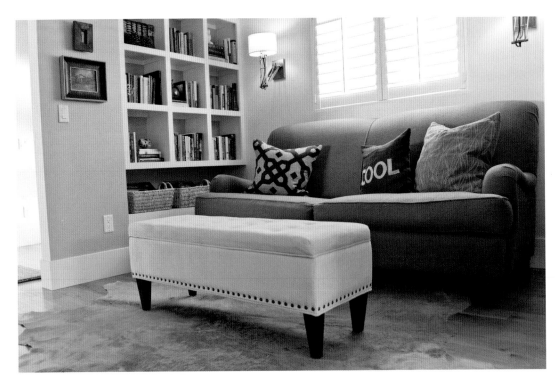

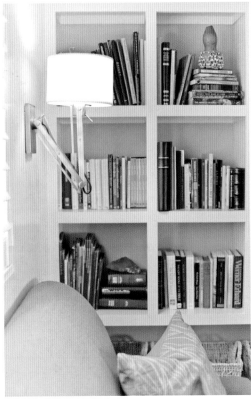

THE LEISURELY SPACE is distinctly separate from the heart of the home. It serves the entire family in a variety of activities from watching TV to quiet contemplation.

SWING-ARM SCONCES were installed behind the ends of the sofa since the room isn't wide enough to accommodate end tables and lamps.

TYING IT TOGETHER
Elements of a Sanctuary

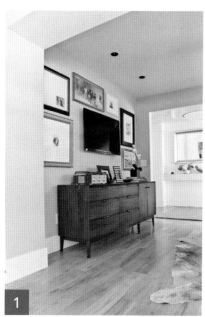
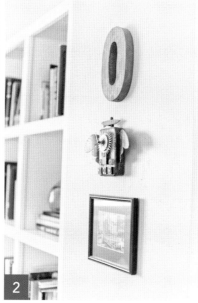
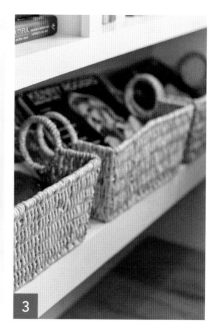

1 A ROOM DESIGNATED as an *in-between space* can also serve another function, such as watching TV.

2 RANDOM YET MEANINGFUL objects and artwork flank the built-in shelving and reflect the Olsens' creative *personality*.

3 DECORATIVE BASKETS are filled with *things that matter*: a lifetime collection of Jeff and Tonya's favorite albums.

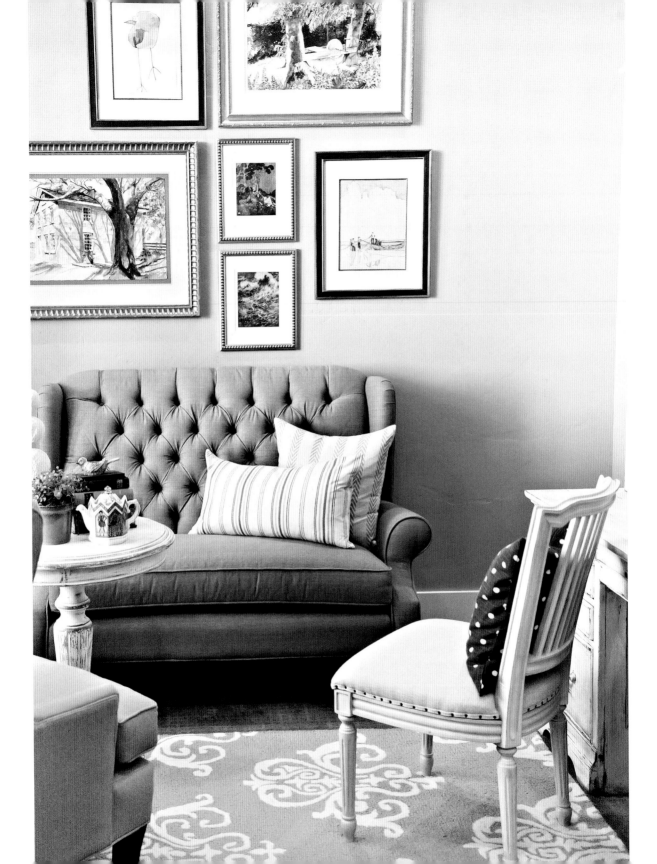

WORK OF ART

When designer Deboni Sacre first arrived at Jan Farris's home for an initial consultation, she was awestruck by Jan's artistic talent. Gorgeous artwork hung throughout the space, inspiring Deboni from the moment she walked in. While Jan inherently understood color theory and design principles, she asked for Deboni's guidance when it came to her new medium, her home.

Instead of hand-holding on every decision, Deboni created a general design plan that allowed Jan to pursue her renovation at her own pace. After a couple of meetings, a few concept images, and a color palette, Jan was equipped to design her home on her own.

Empty nesters, Jan and her husband wanted an open and welcoming place for their grandchildren to visit. A lighter color palette offered a lively departure from the deep greens, rich reds, and muddy browns. Instead, soft grays, creamy golds, and calming blues transformed Jan's home into a welcoming home. The change in color alone was enough to make a dramatic improvement in the space.

Deboni suggested hanging a gallery of meaningful art to serve as daily reminders of family members, travels, and heritage. Jan's personal artwork is intermingled with work from her father and grandchildren. The gallery wall also serves as a focal point in the space. This previously underused room, even with its feminine touch, is now a favorite place for Jan's husband to read and meditate.

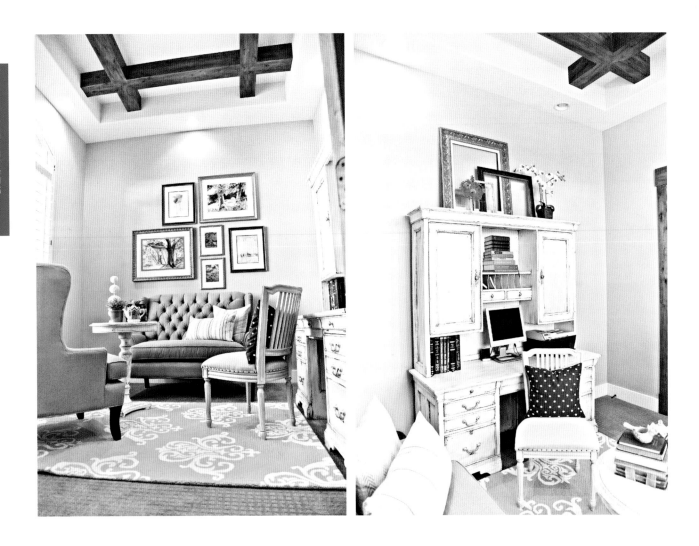

A BROWN COMPUTER DESK gets a facelift with a few coats of warm paint colors. The light gray walls open up the space, making it feel more spacious.

FAUX WOOD BEAMS, stained to match the floor, add visual interest to the ceiling of this small space.

THE NEUTRAL COLOR PALETTE of the room is dramatized by a bright blue pillow and a cheery yellow area rug.

TYING IT TOGETHER

Elements of a Sanctuary

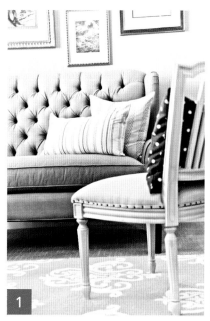

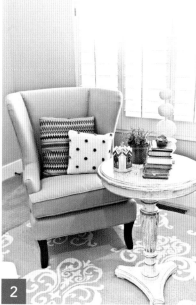

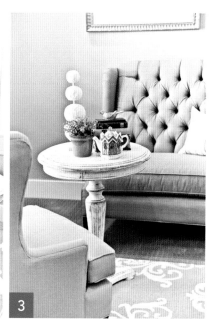

1   A DESK CHAIR serves as extra seating when the room is used as a *gathering space* for friends and family.

2   A SUBTLE COLOR PALETTE lays the foundation and emphasizes the oversized scale of an ochre wing-back chair.

3   A TEA TABLE replaces a bulky coffee table that once filled the room, creating a more comfortable *human scale* in the space.

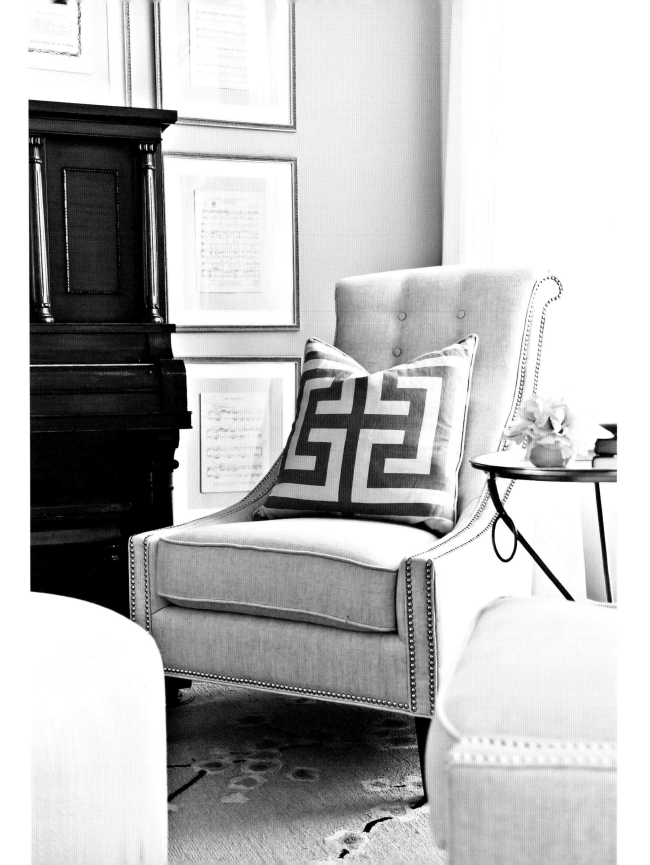

MUSICAL ARRANGEMENT

Shannon Baldwin has a few treasures in her home. The first, and most important, is the one-hundred-plus-year-old Cornish piano, a family heirloom. The other is the room that designer Pamela Jensen designed around the piano, creating a sanctuary that reflects the family heritage.

The piano, originally her great-great-grandmother's, was purchased by Shannon's grandmother, a gifted pianist. It was eventually passed on to Shannon. With it came some of her great-grandmother's sheet music, some of it signed by original composers, with pieces dating back to the 1870s.

Shannon wanted the room to feel serene and have a meditative quality, so she chose a color palette of soft blue, cream, and light gray. Pillows are embellished with a muted persimmon Greek key motif and subtle color. The focal point of the room, however, is the framed sheet music surrounding the piano.

Shannon and her family use the room as a source of inspiration, and the decor helps them remember and appreciate their legacy.

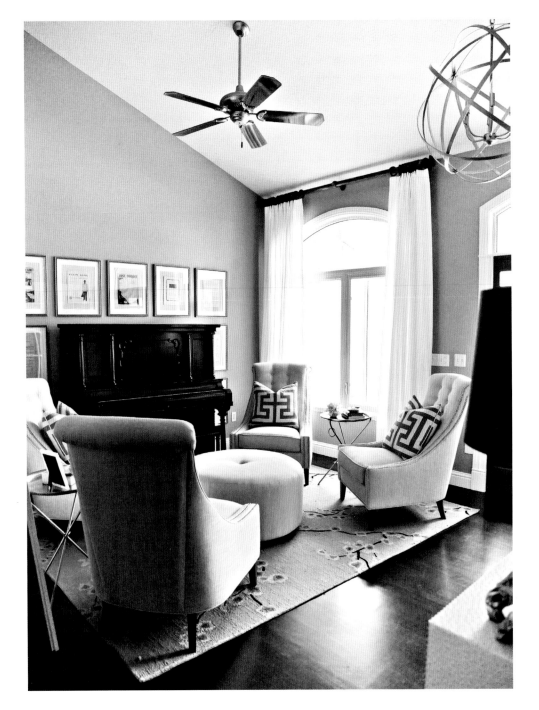

HAVING A PIANO in any space makes a functional seating arrangement more difficult. Pamela chose to place the piano on the focal wall and opted for four chairs surrounding an ottoman to keep the room open.

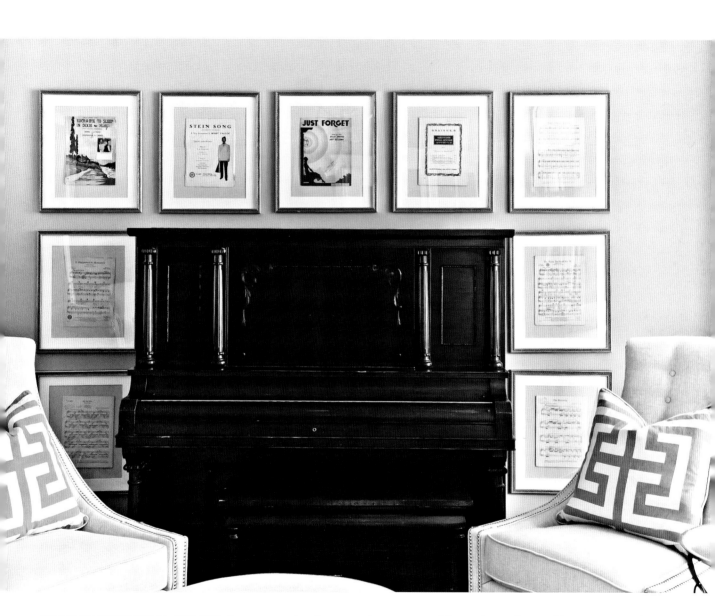

FAMILY HISTORICAL RELICS deserve to be front and center and hang in a place of honor around the piano

PAMELA SELECTED A VIBRANT BLUE for the front door. An area rug helps define the sitting room, which flows in from the entry. .

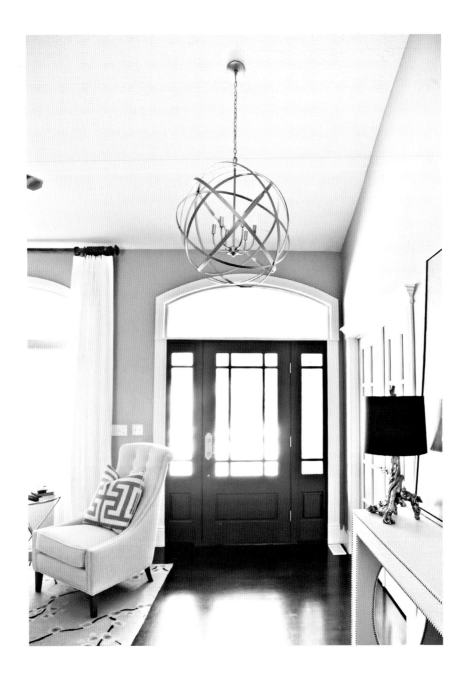

TYING IT TOGETHER

Elements of a Sanctuary

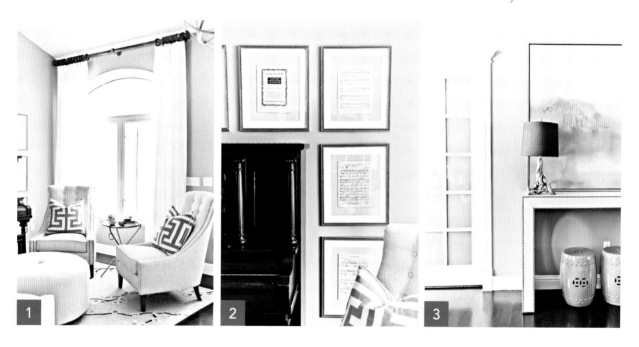

1 DRAPES SOFTEN an oversized arched window, bringing in the *human scale.*

2 THE PIANO and the surrounding framed music from the homeowner's grandmother serves as the room's focal point, a basic *design principle.*

3 ACROSS FROM the sitting room, in the informal entry, apple-green garden stools and cobalt-blue lamps add a touch of Shannon's *personality.*

TYING IT TOGETHER

Elements of a Sanctuary

Connection to Nature

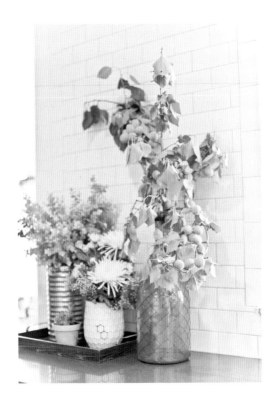

"Nature is the inspiration to all ornamentation."

—Frank Lloyd Wright

CONNECTION TO NATURE

Our inherent connection to nature resonates with each and every one of us on a soul-stirring level. Recently, a significant amount of research has focused on the so-called "nature connection" and how it affects our health, outlook, and overall life. In general, this research shows that the more we can connect with nature and natural elements, the better mental, emotional, and physical health we have.

Look for unique ways to embed nature into your space. This will enhance your life and the lives of others who share your home. Highlight a view. Add natural elements to your decor, such as branches, sea shells, or plants. Open the windows. Listen to the breeze. Experience your senses outdoors. It's good for your all-around health.

Our adrenal systems are in constant overdrive when we are continuously exposed to overstimulating environments. Environments congruent with nature give our minds and bodies an opportunity to relax, ultimately transforming us on a cellular level. Experiencing nature, even at a nominal level, is invigorating to our soul. Nature allows us to slow down and refocus our lives on what really matters.

Patios, sunrooms, porches, and even outdoor kitchens can all be modified for year-round use. Sliding and removable window panels make creating an indoor/outdoor space easier than ever. Furnishing these rooms with durable yet comfortable all-weather furniture makes these spaces the best of both worlds.

Even experiencing nature through the simple view of a window, regardless of the outdoor scene, has a profound effect on our well-being. When natural light infiltrates our system, every fiber of our being is invigorated. Opening windows allows the sounds and smells to further enhance the pleasure of such an experience.

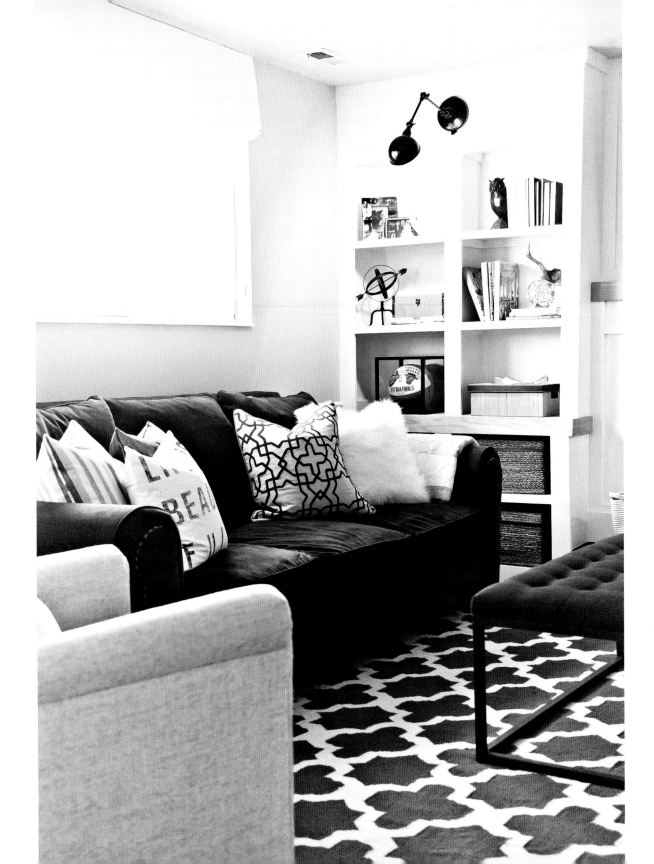

MAJOR STYLE, MINOR BUDGET

Pamela Jensen and her husband, Travis, had their work cut out for them when they moved into their modest yet severely outdated home six years ago. Sky-blue carpet and bunny wallpaper covered the house from top to bottom.

Fortunately, as lead designer at Liv Showroom, Pamela had a vision for her basement family room from the get-go. With a limited budget, she engaged Travis's handyman skills, and together they created a renewed gathering space that fits their lifestyle, connects to nature, and showcases the things they love.

Pamela and Travis wanted plenty of seating for friends and family and room for their puppies and kittens. Pamela designed the space around an oversized pair of chocolate-brown sofas she found that were "too good of a deal to pass up." An upholstered ottoman provides additional seating as well.

Classic navy was selected as an accent color for the room. A geometric magenta area rug adds contrast to rich colors in the room. Travis's nature photography is displayed around the room and shows the couple's love of the outdoors. Built-ins offer a place for storage and order. Library sconces add a classical touch to the top of the cabinets and provide ambient lighting in the room.

Pamela and Travis's love of hunting, fishing, and the outdoors is tastefully woven into their family room, avoiding the stereotypical camouflage theme so often used in rooms related to outdoor activities.

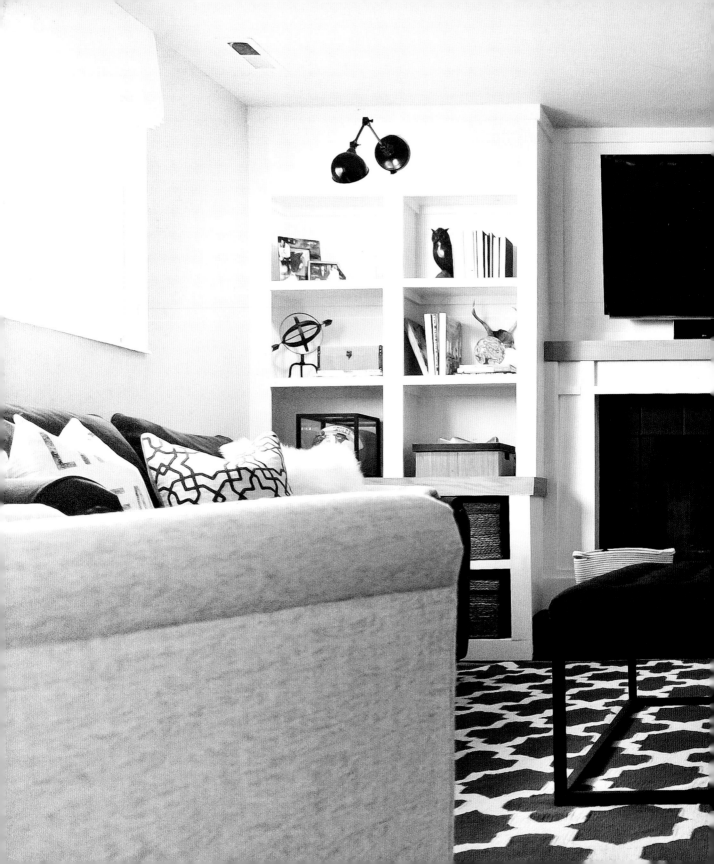

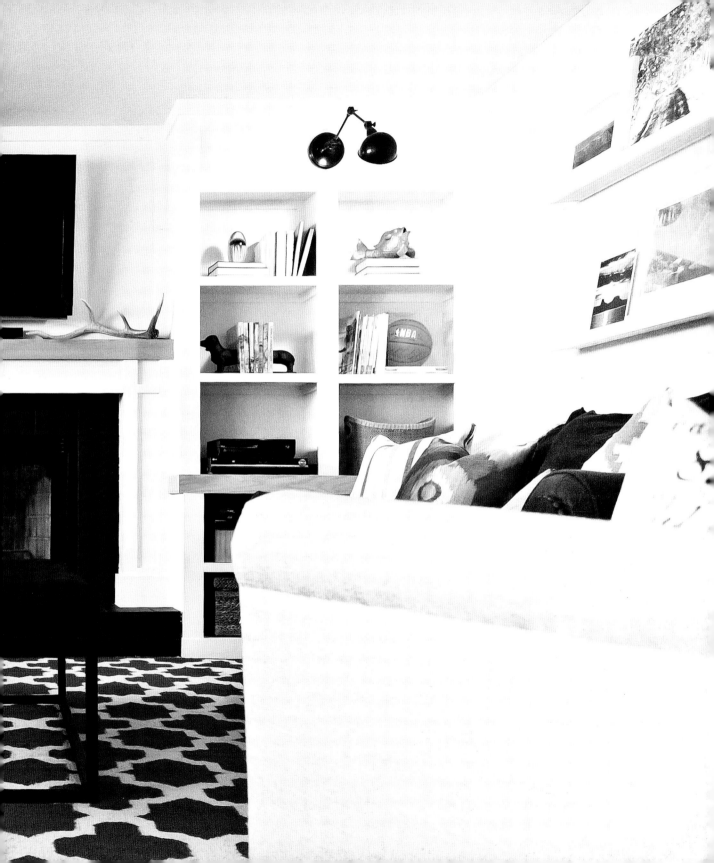

NATURAL LIGHT floods the walk-out basement and creates an expansive feeling in the underground space.

PAM'S DOG Trigger poses in front of the fireplace. The darker colors used throughout the room hide dirt and are pet friendly.

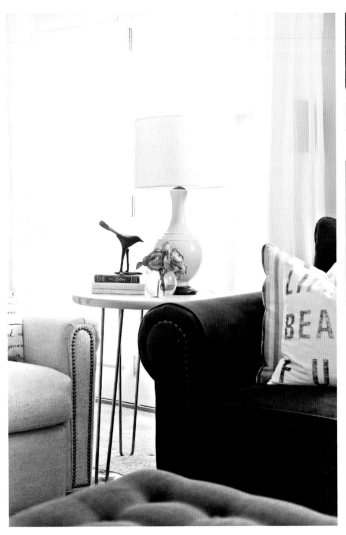

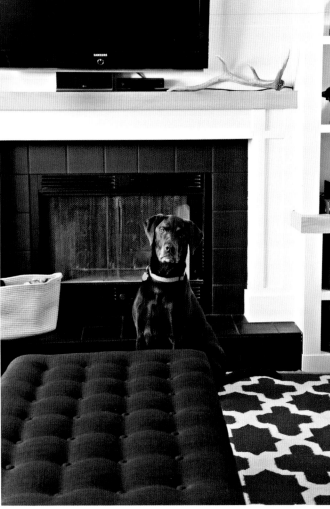

TYING IT TOGETHER

Elements of a Sanctuary

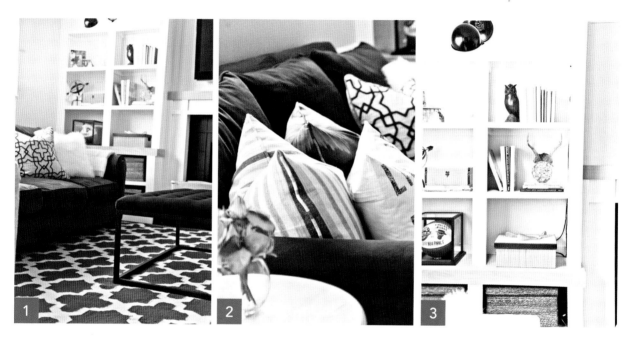

1 SEATING INCLUDES two sofas, two club chairs, and an upholstered ottoman. The *human scale* of these pieces fits well in the small space.

2 DETAILS LIKE a single flower arrangement, cut fresh from the garden, add an element of *nature*.

3 BUILT-IN BOOKSHELVES showcase *things that matter* and baskets provide *order* for unsightly components.

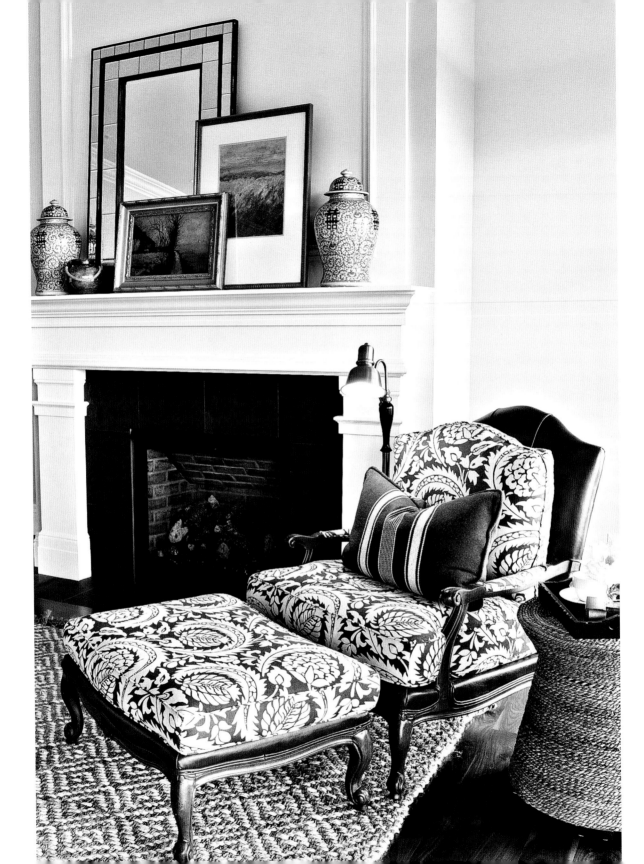

GRAND VIEW

Joyce and Brian Smith built their new home in an established Utah neighborhood in the high hills of the former Bonneville shoreline. The Smiths purchased their property and designed their home to simultaneously maximize views of the city below and the mountainous terrain above.

Joyce's refined taste is apparent in the rich walnut flooring, traditional furnishings, and antique decor. She hired designer Pamela Jensen before construction began to assist in infusing her home with time-honored details and classic style.

Keeping in mind her home's tall ceilings and large floor plan, Pamela worked carefully to ensure all the elements were the appropriate size and scale. A series of large windows and french doors envelop the back of the home from the living room, offering easy access to a secluded patio. Unadorned windows allow plenty of sunlight to embrace the room. The living room combined with the outdoor patio provides plenty of space to gather friends and family in the warmer months when the Smiths entertain.

A dining area isn't tucked away in a hidden room far from the heart of the home. This allows for more use of the gathering space for important family meals together.

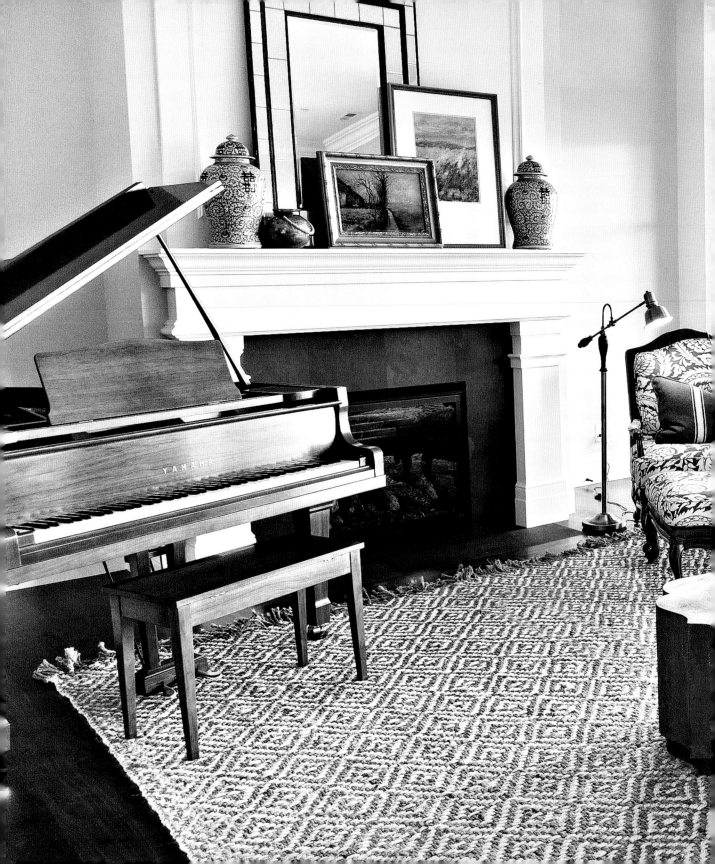

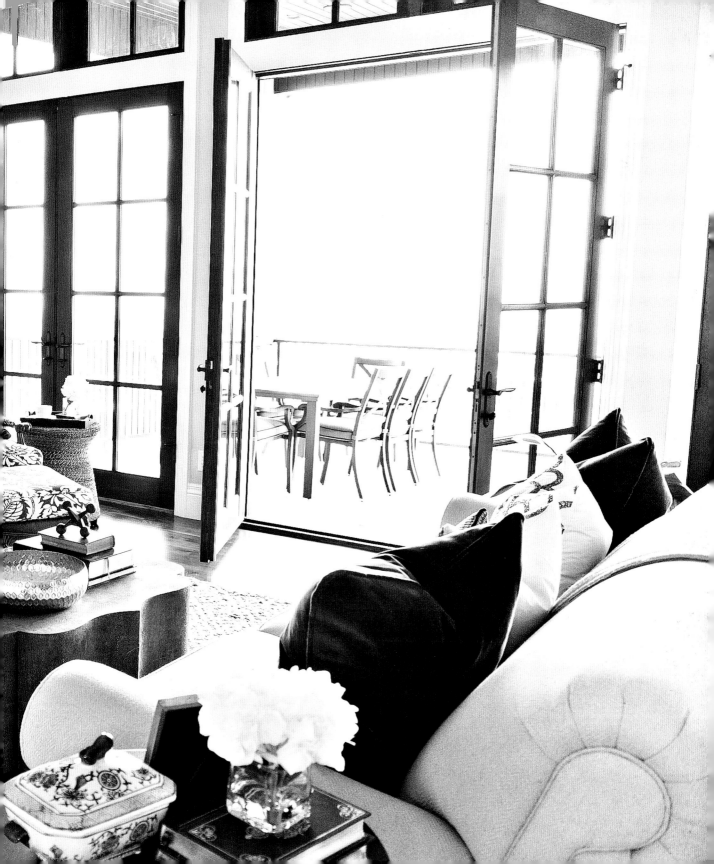

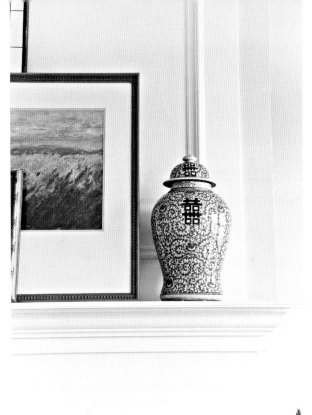

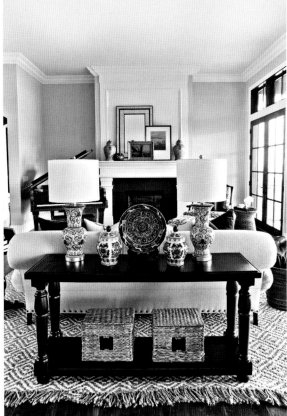

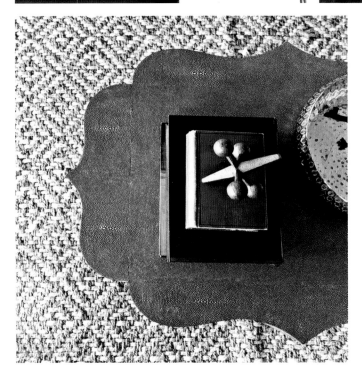

OVERSIZED GINGER JARS flank artwork on the mantel. The artwork is layered to add dimension and interest.

ELEGANT BLUE and white porcelain accents juxtapose the coarse texture of the area rug.

A FAUX SHAGREEN (that's fancy talk for shark skin) coffee table with detailed edging adds texture and an unexpected element.

TYING IT TOGETHER

Elements of a Sanctuary

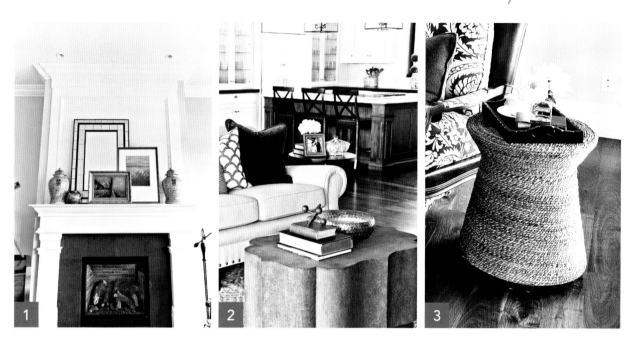

1   THE FLOOR-TO-CEILING fireplace is proportionate to *human scale* in the otherwise grand space. Intricate molding *details* add a refined sense of class.

2   THIS FAMILY ROOM is open to the kitchen, like many modern homes today. Family members can perform their own tasks while still spending time together in this *gathering space*.

3   SMALL DETAILS like this tray and flowers give this room unique charm.

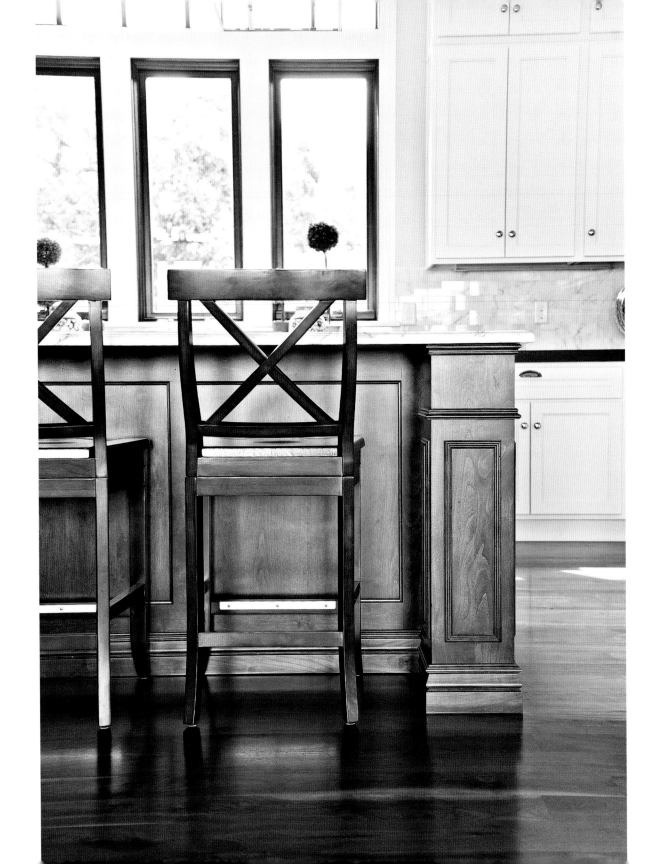

EVERYTHING AND THE KITCHEN SINK

The kitchen is usually the heart of the home, so when Joyce and Brian Smith engaged designer Pamela Jensen to help them with the design details of their new home, they took extra care to create a relaxing space with plenty of room for cooking, eating, and entertaining. The open floor plan flows freely into the adjacent dining and living areas. Although the room itself is formal, Joyce made sure it was comfortable as well.

Pam's main goal was to marry modern function with classic style. Walnut cabinets, Calcutta marble, and creamy white cabinets create a sense of timeless elegance. Large, austere windows, encased by upper cabinets, grace the front of the kitchen, offering up views of the majestic mountainside. An oversized island anchors the expansive space and provides a natural gathering space for friends and family. Glass-front cabinets bring an element of beauty next to a paneled refrigerator. Pamela added simple columns to the base cabinets to create a furniture-like feel. Vintage lanterns illuminate the marble-topped island. Lofty ceilings are visually drawn down with ceiling-height cabinets. Extra storage above is easily accessible with a stool.

Joyce and her family enjoy spending time in their kitchen, and that's just the way they planned it.

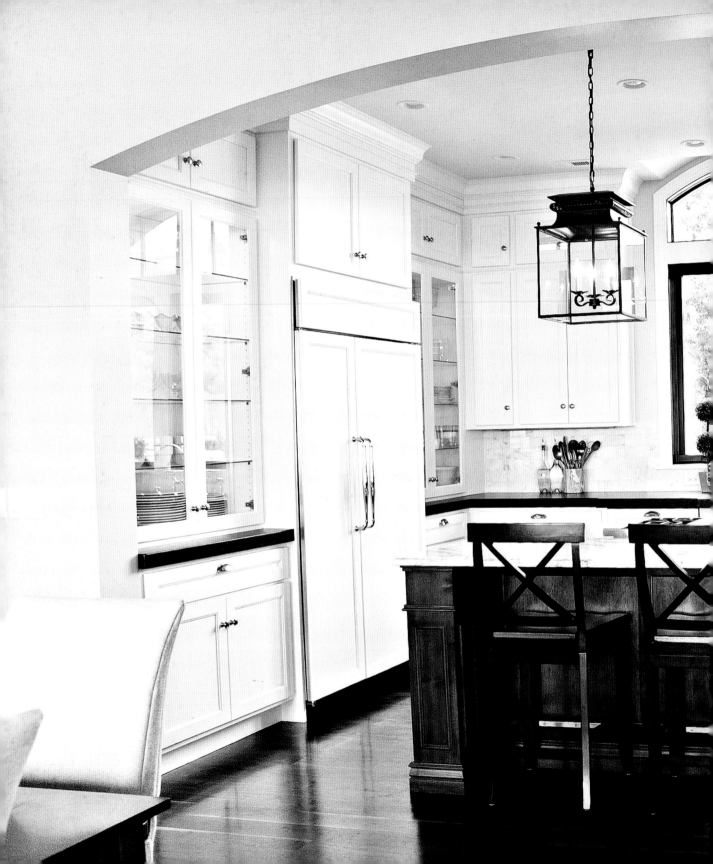

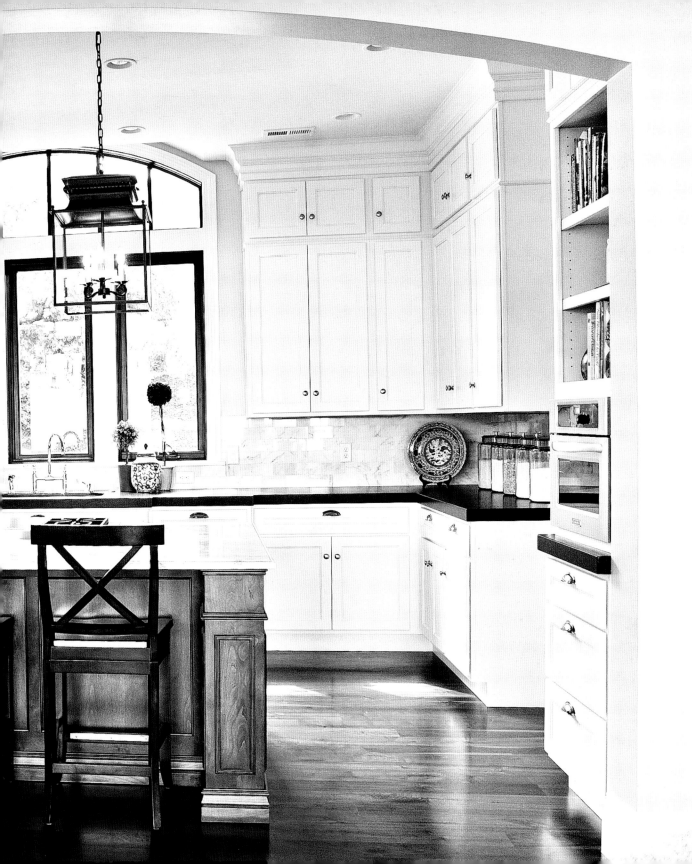

IN CONTRAST to the dark floors, the cabinets were painted a creamy white. The island was stained to match the floors and creates visual weight in the center of the spacious room.

MEAL PREPARATION and dish washing are certainly more enjoyable with gorgeous views in this mountainside home. Blue and white porcelain ware adds a touch of elegance throughout the space.

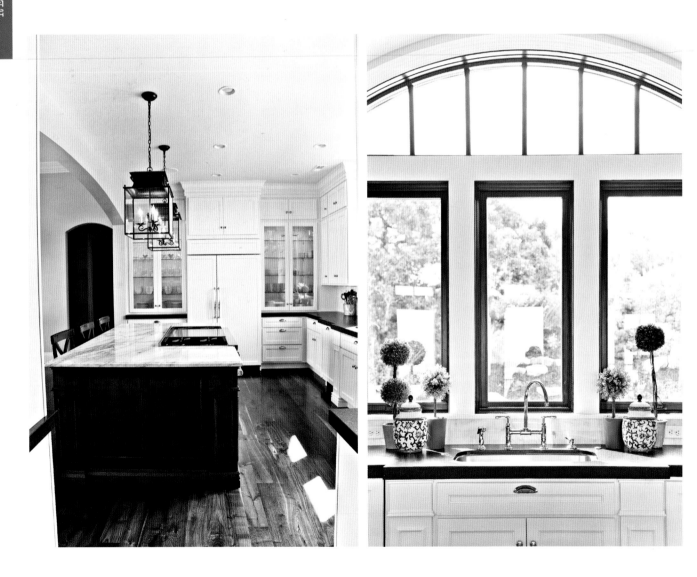

TYING IT TOGETHER

Elements of a Sanctuary

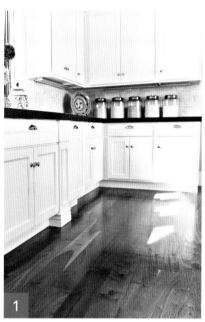
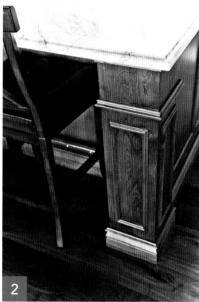
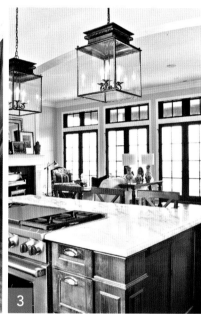

1 ORDER IS MAINTAINED with an abundance of elegant storage.

2 CHUNKY COLUMNS were chosen to add mass and *detail* to the island.

3 COOKING IN THIS KITCHEN is never lonely and creates a great *gathering space* when combined with the adjoining family and dining areas.

CREDITS

We would like to give our heartfelt thanks to the following for letting us feature your beautiful sanctuaries in our book:

Jeff, Shannon, and Brooklyn Baldwin

Brad and Teresa Call

Randy and Kassi Capener

Larry and Jan Farris

Joseph and Kristy Feller

Travis and Pamela Jensen

Randon and Cami Jensen

Matt and Amy Johnson

Tim, Christine, and Kayla Krstic

Dan and Heidi Lowe

Rachelle and Kyle Olsen

Jeff and Tonya Olsen

Christy Petrie

Lori Radman

Rainey Homes

Laurie Riedinger

Russell and Deboni Sacre

Brian and Joyce Smith

Brent and Lisa Taggart

Zeke and Samantha Zenger

RESOURCES

FABRIC/TEXTILES

Caitlin Wilson Design	caitlinwilsontextiles.com
Duralee	duralee.com
DwellStudio	dwellstudio.com
Fabricut	fabricut.com
Kravet	kravet.com
Lacefield Designs	lacefielddesigns.com
Maxwell Fabrics	maxwellfabrics.com
Priemer Prints, Inc.	premierprintsinc.com
The Robert Allen Group	robertallendesign.com
Romo	romo.com
Samuel & Sons	samuelandsons.com
Seabrook	seabrookwallpaper.com
Thibaut	thibautdesign.com
Thomas Paul	shopthomaspaul.com
Classic Home	classichomefurnishings.com

UPHOLSTERY & CASEGOODS

Arteriors	arteriorshome.com
Bliss Studio	blissstudio.com
Blue Ocean Traders	blueoceantraders.com
The Bramble Company	brambleco.com
Brownstone Upholstery	www.brownstoneupholstery.com
Butler Specialty Company	butlerspecialtyfurniture.net
Caracole	caracole.com
Classic Home	classichomefurnishings.com
Crate and Barrel	crateandbarrel.com
Dovetail	dovetailfurniture.info
Foreside Home and Garden	foresidehomeandgarden.com
Four Hands	fourhands.com

Gabby	gabbyhome.com
GO Home Ltd.	gohomeltd.com
GuildMaster	guildmaster.com
Madera Home	maderahomefurniture.com
Noir	noirfurniturela.com
Norwalk	norwalkfurniture.com
Oly Studio	olystudio.com
Orient Express Furniture	orientexpressfurniture.com
Sarreid Ltd.	sarreid.com
Schnadig	schnadig.com
Southfield Furniture	southfieldfurniture.net
Stanley Furniture	stanleyfurniture.com
Sunpan	sunpan.com
Worlds Away	worlds-away.com

WINDOW COVERINGS

Brimar	brimarinc.com
Fabricut	fabricut.com
Quality Curtain Hardware	qualitycurtainhardware.com
Superior Roman Shades	superiorshades.com
Windows West	windowswest.com

ARTWORK

Wendover Art Group	wendoverart.com
Leftbank Art	leftbankart.com
Soicher Marin	soicher-marin.com

ACCESSORIES

Arteriors	arteriorshome.com
Creative Co-Op	creativecoop.com
Cyan Design	cyandesign.biz
Dash & Albert	dashandalbert.com
Global Views	globalviews.com
HomArt	homart.com

International Handicrafts, Inc.　ihionline.com
Legend of Asia　legendofasia.net
Silks Are Forever　silksareforever.com
StyleCraft　stylecraftonline.com
Import Collection　importcollection.com
The Light Garden　thelightgarden.com
Two's Company/Tozai　twoscompany.com

LIGHTING

AFLighting　aflighting.com
Arteriors　arteriorshome.com
Barn Light Electric　barnlightelectric.com
Currey & Company　curreycodealers.com
Lamps Plus　lampsplus.com
Robert Abbey　robertabbey.com
StyleCraft　stylecraftonline.com
Visual Comfort　visualcomfort.com

CARPET/RUGS

Capel Rugs　capelrugs.com
Jaipur Rugs　jaipurrugs.com
Robertex　robertex.com
Shaw Contract Group　shawcontract.com
Surya　surya.com
Unique Carpets, Ltd.　uniquecarpetsltd.com

WALLPAPER

Graham & Brown　grahamandbrown.com
Koroseal Interior Products　koroseal.com
Romo　romo.com
Seabrook Wallpaper　seabrookwallpaper.com
Thibaut　thibautdesign.com

RESOURCES

TILE/STONE

ANN SACKS	annsacks.com
Arizona Tile	arizonatile.com
Contempo Tile & Stone	contempotile.com
Daltile	daltile.com
Emser Tile	emser.com
European Marble & Granite	europeanmarbleandgranite.net
Marazzi USA	marazziusa.com
Old World Stone Imports	oldworldstoneimports.com

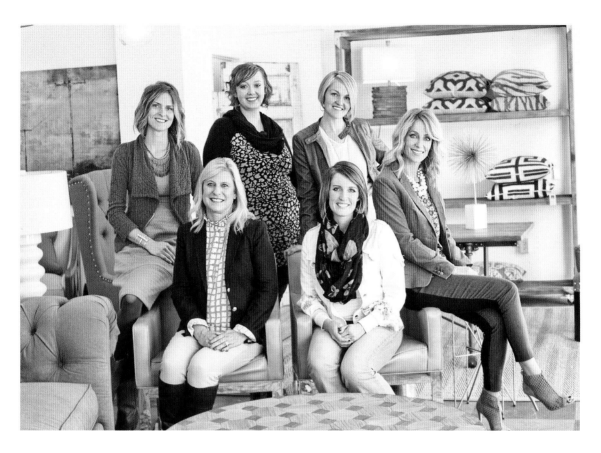

ABOUT THE TEAM

People are sometimes nervous about engaging an interior designer. Because we're so—you know—something. We get that. But at Liv Showroom, we feel like we're a bit different. Talk to us and you'll find we know our stuff, but you'll also find we're a lot like you. We know that spaces need to be livable and not overly precious. Every project is a new opportunity for our team of creative experts to transform environments from ordinary to extraordinary.

Liv Showroom is a full-service interior design firm and showroom. Our retail location and design studio is located on historic Main Street in Bountiful, Utah.

Our team as pictured from left to right: BACK—Samantha Zenger, Pamela Jensen, Deboni Sacre, and Tonya Olsen. FRONT—Kristen Holm and Jenny Butler.

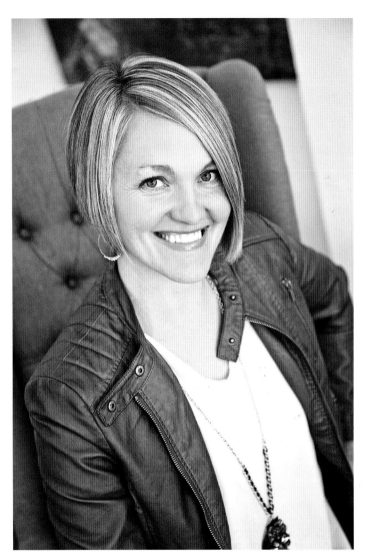

ABOUT THE AUTHOR

DEBONI SACRE has known her life's mission to create inspiring and timeless interiors since childhood. Her passion for design stems from a firm belief that beauty is a positive force. She enjoys the challenge of creating unique environments that brings both function and joy to her clients and their families.

Shortly after completing her design degree in 2005, Deboni opened a full-service interior design firm, which eventually became Liv Showroom. Later, she expanded to a retail showroom in Bountiful, Utah, where she loves working closely with the other talented designers and staff. Deboni is grateful for her trusting and loyal clients who have allowed her to explore her lifetime passion for the past fourteen years.

Deboni loves where she lives in Stansbury Park, Utah, with her husband and four children. She values her role of motherhood most of all.

ABOUT THE AUTHOR

TONYA OLSEN has always had a passion for designing timeless, charming interiors. She loves working intimately with each client to create functional and creative spaces that reflect their unique personalities. Her amazing attention to detail has led to her notable reputation with clients, contractors, and building partners alike.

Tonya shares ownership of Liv Showroom, a full-service interior design firm and retail showroom, and holds a master's degree in interior design. Tonya has been featured on many morning talk shows, blogs, magazines, and more.

Tonya has a lifetime of personal adventures in interior design and over twenty years of professional design experience. She is the author of *Room Recipes: A Creative and Stylish Guide to Interior Design*. Tonya, her husband, and their three boys have created their personal sanctuary in Bountiful, Utah.

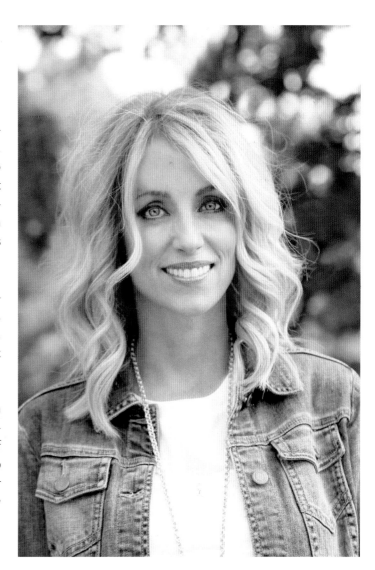

TONYA OLSEN

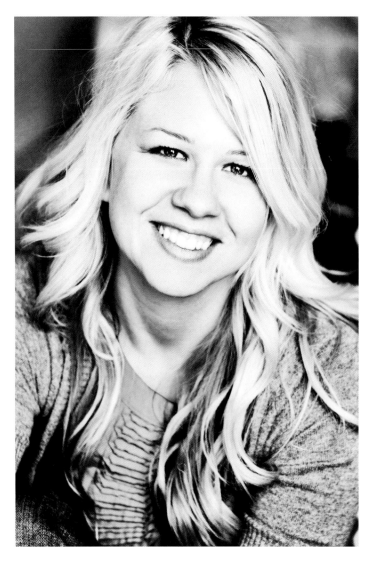

ABOUT THE PHOTOGRAPHER

SARA BOULTER is a photographer based in Salt Lake City, Utah. When she's not photographing drool-worthy homes or beautiful brides, Sara can be found spending time with her family, daydreaming about interior design, traveling the globe, snuggling an animal, or feeding her Instagram addiction. Visit her at www.saraboulterphotography.com.